How the Weather Affects Your Health

...gives you the awareness that your environment, in this case the weather, has a much greater impact on your wellbeing than any of us would like to admit. ...It is only a small step towards the awareness that everything in nature is connected.

How the Weather Affects Your Health

Manfred Kaiser

New Age Books

ISBN: 978-81-7822-320-9

First Indian Edition: 2009

First published in Australia 2002 by
Michelle Anderson Publishing Pty Ltd., Melbourne 3000

Published by
NEW AGE BOOKS
A-44 Naraina Phase-I
New Delhi-110 028 (INDIA)
Email: nab@vsnl.in
Website: www.newagebooksindia.com

For Sale in India Only

Printed in India
at Shri Jainendra Press
A-45 Naraina Phase-I, New Delhi-110 028

Contents

Introduction

The weather and our health are on our lips more often than we probably realize: 'The heat is killing me. I can't stand the cold. This wind is driving me crazy.' When we are short of a topic for a conversation, we talk about the weather and its myriad ill effects. A survey conducted by the Internet site for *The Weather Channel* also found that over 70% of Americans believe the weather influences their wellbeing. So why is it that we know instinctively when weather affects us? Why doesn't science want to know? Where can you find more information?

When a heat wave kills hundreds of elderly people or the skin cancer rate increases dramatically, health authorities begin initiatives to educate the public. They advise on the dangers of extreme heat and ultraviolet (UV) radiation. Sadly, and despite mounting evidence that weather has a profound impact on our health, this is where a lot of people's understanding ends.

> 'Scientists know a lot about things you are not interested in, but don't know much about the things you want to know.' (Unknown)

Try the library, or newspapers, magazines, journals and the Internet. Yes the information is there, but quite widely scattered and often hidden in jargon that nobody can understand. *How the Weather Affects Your Health*, however, compiles the vast information from many fields of science into one easy-to-read work. It provides you with the knowledge to link certain symptoms with certain weather conditions. If you suffer from headache or migraine, you may find that a dry wind, approaching weather front or charged atmosphere is the trigger for your ordeal. You'll be able to explain why your rheumatic back hurts most when the weather changes, and take steps to prevent or alleviate the pain.

How the Weather Affects Your Health also explains that even the air we breathe is never pure, that natural and man-made impurities exist in every corner of the world and lead to health problems. Wind can carry largely undiluted pollution for hundreds of kilometres and dump the toxins upon unsuspecting populations. Air impurities trigger dreadful symptoms amongst an ever-increasing number of hay fever and asthma sufferers. Some tiny particles penetrate deep into the lungs and enter the bloodstream, and scientists link them with heart and circulatory disorders.

You will learn how your body regulates its temperature and how you adapt to outside temperature changes. Whenever your body temperature climbs or drops beyond a certain level, health problems occur—they can be just swollen legs during hot conditions, or deadly hypothermia after cold exposure. Temperature extremes influence human well-being most and take the blame for high mortality rates.

Most people know that UV radiation burns the skin and may cause skin cancer. Some are aware of other illnesses or problems associated with sunlight. Less people know that UV radiation ages the skin, degenerates eyesight and inhibits the body's immune system. And how many people really believe that a lack of sunlight is a major cause for mood swings and depressions?

> 'A new danger is the transfer of infective organisms between the animal kingdom and the alarming potential of environmental changes with their serious effects on health.'
>
> '. . . the present severe weather conditions in [the UK] are, I have no doubt, the consequences of mankind's arrogant disregard of the delicate balance of Nature.'
>
> (Prince Charles in his speech to the British Medical Association's Millennium Festival of Medicine in November 2000.)

How the Weather Affects Your Health explains the creation of wind, flood and lightning events and their detrimental effects on society. We've all noticed that the frequency and severity of extreme weather events have increased in recent years. Scientists still debate whether global warming or a natural cycle is the cause. Whatever the reason, severe storms, lightning and floods cause thousands of deaths and billions of dollars worth of damage worldwide. Dr Gro Harlem Brundtland, Director-General of the World Health Organisation, highlighted some of the challenges facing the global community in his speech on World Meteorological Day in Geneva in 1999:

'... We have evidence to state that climate change—by altering weather patterns and by disturbing life-supporting natural systems and processes—affects the health of human populations. There are many effects of these changes. And there is still discussion on the exact causality between human behaviour and climate change. But we know enough to take this very seriously and we have every reason to be concerned about adverse consequences for human health. The world's climate is warming and we know that human behaviour has a role in that phenomenon through the sharply increasing emission of greenhouse gases. We must expect that this trend, if continued, will have profound consequences for life on Earth and for the health of human beings. What can be done to meet these profound challenges?

At the outset we need to revert to the broader agenda of sustainable development. The message of Our Common Future—reiterated at Rio—was the link between environment and development. We called for a new era of economic growth—growth that is forceful and at the same time socially and environmentally sustainable. In that process the developed countries must show their share of solidarity. Poverty is in itself the prime polluter. Populations have a right to lift themselves out of poverty. The developed world cannot pull up the ladder and say: sorry—we filled the waste baskets—there is no room left for you. We need to continue the work to take the Climate convention further—step by step—based on evidence, and new mechanisms of burden sharing.'

Today, the public is no longer content with scientific medical explanations for their health problems—the rapid rise in popularity of alternative medicine and therapies proves this. Awareness is growing that humans are part of nature, and that the environment is controlling their wellbeing. Weather services around the world are catching up with this public trend and issue bioweather forecasts for UV radiation, air quality and pollen concentrations. Some go further and warn migraine sufferers, heart patients and people with asthma of certain weather changes.

How the Weather Affects Your Health is not a medical self-help book. You will find tips on treatment and prevention, but they are only there as information and should not replace sound medical advice. Nevertheless, knowledge of the effects of certain weather conditions allows you to prepare for them and avoid circumstances that may lead to health problems.

chapter one

Bioweather

What is bioweather?

High up in the atmosphere, the weather is rather boring. Above eight kilometres at the poles, and 16 km at the equator, nothing much happens, as airline pilots know. For the sake of your stomach, and to save cleaning staff wages, they climb to levels where the winds are more or less steady—no ups and downs. The joy lasts for only a few hours, though. Eventually and despite the complimentary food and drinks, you have to land somewhere. At the destination, the pilot descends through the often tumultuous few kilometres just above the earth's surface. Now we talk weather.

Weather is the state of the atmosphere at a particular location and at a particular time. Observers measure, record and report the changes. They describe the situation with expressions such as cloudy, fine, rainy or windy, and use measurements to determine temperature, humidity, air pressure, precipitation and wind speed. Certain weather conditions that get on your nerves or make you sick, however, are called bioweather: the wind that comes down the mountain range gives you a migraine, the terrible heat makes your blood boil, an old wound starts to itch. No, the ups and downs during flight aren't bioweather, no matter how sick you feel.

Bioweather follows your life from conception to the grave. The weather influenced the time your mother became pregnant and determined your birthday. The weather will very likely control the day you part with life while, in the meantime, your bioweather makes you moody or sick.

Nowadays you can find bioweather forecasts next to the 'ordinary' weather in all major news media. The predictions are simple UV indexes for the next day, smog alerts or pollen warnings. They can be quite elaborate and include indexes for mood, labour and birth, or alertness.

Bioweather is sometimes referred to as bioclimate. Both terms are probably meant in the same sense but describe different situations. Climate is the average weather over a length of time. For example, if a climatologist adds up all recorded values for a particular month or year and calculates the average, then he or she can describe the climate of a town or a region. Of course, a month or a year is not enough to give a true picture. The climatologist requires years of weather recordings to give a reasonable reflection of the climate.

The word climate immediately brings 'change' to mind. The newspapers regularly print articles concerning the possible effects of climate change. There's no doubt that the earth is warming, but should you bother about a rise of less than one degree? You should, because to change a hundred-year average by such a small amount requires much larger short-term fluctuations. In other words, temperature increases have to be significant to impact on a hundred-year average.

Medicine and bioweather

'Whoever wishes to investigate medicine properly, should proceed thus: in the first place to consider the seasons of the year, and what effects each of them produces for they are not at all alike, but differ much from themselves in regard to their changes. Then the winds, the hot and the cold, especially such as are common to all countries, and then such as are peculiar to each locality.

'For if one knows all these things well, or at least the greater part of them, he cannot miss knowing, when he comes into a strange city, either the diseases peculiar to the place, or the particular nature of common diseases, or commit mistakes, as is likely to be the case provided one had not previously considered these matters.'

These are the words of the ancient Greek physician Hippocrates (460–377 BC). In his famous medical works, he established the connection between human health and environmental factors. Hippocrates and other thinkers of his time discarded magic and religion as cause and cure, and established the practice of clinical medicine. 'Every disease has its own nature, and arises from external causes,' he wrote.

For centuries, medicine drifted away from these beliefs. Medical scientists did seek simple answers to their questions. In the 17th century, the French philosopher René Descartes went so far as to suggest that the human body is a machine and its functions were mechanical. Replace the worn parts, change the oil, lubricate the joints, and detail clean—sure!

While this thought was soon dismissed, it illustrates the 'can-do' attitude of modern science. The medical profession and health authorities are still reluctant to give advice that is based on non-scientific evidence. Today, not one week passes without an announcement of another medical cure. Months or years later, however, this cure may prove to have restrictive side effects and is discarded—quietly, if possible.

Many patients are also sucked into this vortex of medical breakthroughs. They expect or demand a prescription for the miracle drug. Some even change their medical practitioner if he or she suggests an alternative method to treat the cause, thinking that their doctor must be incompetent if they recommend rest instead of the super drug.

This thinking, however, is slowly changing. Patients turn more and more to the traditional or alternative methods of medicine. A growing number of people today lobby the medical profession to consider the benefits of natural remedies. It took the recent boom in the use of natural remedies to shake health authorities and the industry into action. Suddenly, money is available to research the so-called 'folk medicine'.

Patients often know or suspect that certain weather conditions influence their wellbeing. Communicating their knowledge or suspicion to their doctor can be difficult, though. They fear to be branded misguided, or the doctor dismisses their suggestions out of ignorance. Health professionals are fully aware of most heat and cold-related illnesses and know of the ill effects of UV radiation or air pollution. Many, however, don't relate changes in atmospheric conditions to migraine or see the danger to heart patients. Many aren't aware that some types of depression are related to a lack of sunlight and can be treated with artificial light instead of antidepressants.

Once the weather-health connection becomes adequately researched and publicized, you as a patient will be encouraged to tell your doctor of the symptoms you encounter during certain weather conditions. While your doctor can't change the weather for you, he or she will then be able to give you appropriate advice. If drugs are required, you may get away with taking them only in advance of your bioweather.

Bioweather forecasting

A few weather services employ meteorologists with the skill to forecast bioweather. Well-funded national services even allocate scientists to full-time research into this subject. The services offer bioweather forecasts in the same manner as other specialized weather predictions, such as aviation and agriculture forecasts. Radio, T.V, Internet and phone services warn the public of weather and environmental situations that increase pain, trigger medical conditions or are simply uncomfortable. Sufferers of weather-sensitive disorders, such as migraine, rheumatism, asthma, bronchitis, heart and circulatory disorders, can therefore take precautions.

UV radiation reports and forecasts

During the summer months, there is hardly a weather forecast that doesn't have a UV radiation warning attached to it. Health officials in all countries have long warned their residents that too much sunshine can lead to skin cancer, eye problems or immune system disorders. Despite this, many people with fair complexions still believe that a change to bronze or brown is fashionable and depicts general health. But, even if you take precautions, you won't completely escape the ever-increasing amount of harmful radiation. The depleted ozone layer in the upper atmosphere allows more harmful radiation to reach your skin.

Parts of the world have very high rates of skin cancer, and health officials in these regions are therefore particularly vigilant. Meteorological offices issue daily bulletins concerning expected UV radiation levels. They are shown either on maps or in numeric values. With the help of computer models, the forecaster calculates the expected level of radiation that will reach the ground under a cloudless sky. He or she then takes into consideration the date, latitude, cloud cover, altitude and haziness of the air, and converts these factors into an internationally recognized intensity index and issues forecasts for particular locations.

UV Radiation Index

UV Index	Danger Category	Sunsmart Information by the Australian Cancer Society
Below 3	Moderate	Moderate UV levels can still be present when it is cold—like on snowfields. Remember sun-smart habits when you hit the slopes.
3 to 6	High	If UV levels are high most people can get a nasty dose of sunburn even when the temperature is below 27°C.
7 to 9	Very High	UV radiation can still be very high on days when there are clouds. Don't be fooled by cloudy skies.
Above 9	Extreme	Extreme UV radiation can cause unprotected skin to burn after just 12 minutes.

Australian Cancer Society

Air quality reports

Pollution makes you sick and can kill you. People are well aware of that fact and demand action from their governments. Our representatives like to be seen to do something about this menace. But pollution-generating industry argues that drastic measures to curb pollution lead to higher unemployment, negative growth and relocation to places with less stringent regulations. Governments, therefore, establish environmental protection agencies to monitor industry and enforce some pollution reduction laws.

The public also wishes to be informed of pollution levels in their cities and countryside. You can hear smog alerts and air quality reports quite regularly on radio and TV, or read the warnings, analyses and statistics in newspapers or on the Internet.

Unfortunately, nations have adopted different air quality standards to express the level of pollution, whereby a moderate level of pollution in one country would be considered a high level in another. Some countries still deny that pollution exists or is a health hazard.

Environmental agencies issue reports and forecasts on all major pollutants: sulphur dioxide, carbon monoxide, nitrogen oxide, ozone and particulate matter (solid airborne particles). A smog alert or report warns of the combined level of some or all pollutants.

Respiratory distress forecasts

Air pollution isn't the only torment that sufferers with respiratory problems have to endure. Rapid changes in air pressure and temperature can equally trigger bronchial spasms or asthma attacks. Dry gusty winds often dislodge a significant amount of dust particles from the soil, which can then further irritate the airways and lungs. This forecast warns of such conditions.

Pollen concentration

It's easy to find out when the oak tree is in bloom. It is not so easy to predict the pollen concentration for the following day. Certain weather conditions will either hinder or aid the deployment of pollen: without wind the pollen can't get airborne; strong wind will blow the pollen away; moderate wind leads to an increase in pollen concentration; updraughts lift the pollen high into the atmosphere where they catch the prevailing winds; an approaching weather front with rain and lightning increases the amount of allergens in the air; continuous rain will wash the atmosphere clean.

To issue an allergy warning for a region, the forecaster has to predict the weather condition for the following day first. The forecaster then takes into consideration the types of plants in bloom and previous pollen counts.

Extreme temperature forecasts

You don't have to be a weather-sensitive person to suffer from extreme cold or heat. Without doubt, either condition impacts strongly on your wellbeing. In many cases, a cold snap or a heat wave will lead to illness and death. Meteorological forecasters and health professionals therefore issue temperature warnings and give advice to minimize the risk.

A strong wind will increase your sense of cold, and high humidity will increase your sense of heat, so indexes were developed to compensate for the additional influences. Some of these formulas are quite elaborate, and contain factors such as wind, humidity, sun radiation, cloud cover, and the season. A temperature forecast, therefore, can include two values: the actual expected temperature and the apparent temperature. For example: your city expects a temperature of 30°C, but a forecasted humidity of 80% will make you 'feel' a much higher temperature of around 38°C.

Influenza reports

Influenza viruses constantly mutate, often making vaccination programmes ineffective. The flu is, therefore, still a major cause of death and serious illness each year. The World Health Organization (WHO), together with 110 influenza centres in 82 countries, keeps a global watch on influenza outbreaks. The WHO publishes weekly reports of influenza activity and recommendations on the FluNet web site. National health authorities work together with hospitals and professionals to obtain information on the spread of a particular influenza virus. In winter, they release regular reports and warnings.

INFLUENZA SUMMARY UPDATE

(Week ending March 10, 2001 – Week 10)

During Week 10 (March 4–10, 2001), 6% of the specimens tested by WHO and NREVSS laboratories were positive for influenza. The proportion of patient visits to sentinel physicians for influenza-like illness was within baseline levels of 0% to 3% in the United States overall and in 8 of 9 surveillance regions. The proportion of deaths attributed to pneumonia and influenza was 8.0%. This percentage is below the epidemic threshold for this time of year. One state and territorial health department reported widespread influenza activity, 12 reported regional influenza activity, 35 reported sporadic activity, and one reported no influenza activity.

For the current season, the overall national percentage of respiratory specimens positive for influenza appears to have peaked at 24% at the end of January (Week 4). During the past 3 seasons, the peak percentages of respiratory specimens positive for influenza viruses have ranged from 28% to 33%. For this season, the percentage of patient visits to sentinel physicians for influenza-like illness appears to have peaked at 4% in mid to late January. During the past 3 seasons, the peak percentages for such visits ranged between 5% and 6%.

US Centers for Disease Control and Prevention

Other forecasts and reports

Bursts of cold and humid weather swells the old joints painfully. Rapid changes in air pressure trigger migraine in weather-sensitive persons. Wouldn't you like to be forewarned? An **Aches and Pain Forecast** warns of pending weather situations likely to trigger painful symptoms in weather-sensitive individuals.

Your brain appears to function best during periods of high pressure and comfortable temperature and humidity. It is sluggish when heat or extreme cold stresses your body. This assumption forms the basis for a **Mental Alertness and Reaction Time Forecast**.

Statistics prove that a significant fall in air pressure induces labour. A **Labour and Birth** forecast map shows areas with expected rapid falls in air pressure.

Yesterday, a bioweather forecast predicted an overcast sky, misty air and rain. 'That's why I feel so grumpy today,' you say after looking at the **Mood Index**. Strong dry winds will have a similar effect on you.

BIOMETEOROLOGY

What is biometeorology?

Bioweather is the atmospheric condition that influences your wellbeing. Biometeorology is the science that tries to explain why. Advances in statistical mathematics helped confirm the connection between weather and human health, but don't explain why a particular disease proliferates during a particular season, nor why the mortality rate is higher during certain weather events. Some scientists began to seriously research the subject and, in a number of published studies, provided proof beyond doubt that weather influences human health, mood and behaviour—they created the science of biometeorology.

The human body is complex and researchers realized that medicine alone can't explain all ill effects. Biometeorology is, therefore, a combination of many science disciplines, chiefly meteorology, medicine and biology. Amongst other cooperative ventures, scientists exchanged their findings and broadened their research to include the positive and negative influences of weather on all living organisms—humans, animals and plants.

Even scientists like to be organized, so in 1956, a group of them formed the International Society of Biometeorology (ISB). The Society's main goals are the development of biometeorology and the dissemination of information between its members from a variety of disciplines. The *Journal of Biometeorology* is the voice of researchers, and annual international conferences their trading places.

For many years, however, biometeorology was mostly unknown and not respected as science: 'Air pressure changes a source of headache? You've got to be joking.' Yet, the number of jokers grew steadily and delivered enough proof to convince the public and other colleagues. Today the media distributes biometeorology-based health reports, warnings and forecasts. Biometeorology has practical value and will eventually lead to substantial savings in health care spending.

Research

The collection of statistical evidence is, so far, the dominant practice of research into the weather and health relationship. In the last decade scientists evaluated a significant amount of data and published the results in science journals. A statistical analysis establishes *whether* there is a link between weather and health and *what* the risk factors are. Statistics can find threshold values, such as the maximum temperature at which overheating of the body occurs during sport or work. The data shows the number of people affected by weather events, thus helping health authorities and emergency departments to prepare for the adverse effects of expected weather extremes or disasters. Further research, however, has to find out *how* the meteorological elements (temperature, humidity, air pressure etc.) impact on an organism.

Biometeorological research concerns itself in particular with the:

- Effects on human body functions and the mind—mental development, conception, birth, susceptibility to diseases etc.
- Association of weather and climate with human diseases

- Weather sensitivity
- Effects on human activities, such as work, sport, learning
- Human behaviour
- Therapeutic value of climate
- Indoor climate
- Effects on the economy
- Influence of weather and climate on agriculture, horticulture and aquaculture
- Urban design and architecture
- Environment and global warming.

It is difficult to collect data on these subjects. Government agencies from different countries use different sources of information or do not participate in research at all. Researchers themselves often disagree with a colleague's method of data collection. Public records provide some data on the causes of death. Newspapers, magazines and journals contain a limited number of reports and tables on mortality rates for certain environmental conditions. Even harder to obtain is data on age, sex, race and socio-economic status of the victim or patient. But to aid prevention, research in the factors influencing the onset of diseases should have equal if not higher priority to death rate sampling. The medical profession, therefore, needs to cooperate when researchers try to obtain data on weather-related illnesses or injuries.

A further hurdle in biometeorological research is the lack of definitions on what comprises weather or climate-related deaths or medical conditions. For example, a falling tree branch breaks the leg of a person outdoors during a severe storm. What is the cause of injury: the storm that caused the tree to drop the branch, the branch that was too heavy for the leg, or the careless person? The direct cause of the break is obviously the tree branch. But indirectly the weather and the person are also to blame. Can this injury find its way into statistics on storm-related injuries?

Fortunately, however, some fields of biometeorology that were once in urgent need of research are now well sponsored by industry and government alike. Already they provide some benefits to people's wellbeing.

Climate research is a very important aspect in urban design and architecture. Every time a new building, car park or road is constructed, it alters the climate. The change inflicted by one building or road is minimal, but the effect of towns and cities is significant. The city is warmer than its surroundings and influences wind speed and direction (see 'Heat Island Effect' in Chapter Four, 'Heat'). With a little foresight, and perhaps government legislation, the town planners can minimize the effects of heat waves and flash floods. Clever house designs provide you with a comfortable and energy-efficient home.

Weather and climate as therapy is nothing new. The ancient Greeks and Romans recognized the benefits and recuperated in health spas and resorts. Many countries make prevention of illness an important goal. Government health agencies and insurance companies now see the long-term health benefits to people, and subsidize such therapies. The challenge for research is to develop international guidelines on what constitutes a health resort or spa. It is of not much value if the resort provides massages, baths and healthy activities, but is located downwind of a major industrial area.

chapter two

Weather Sensitivity

Blame weather sensitivity for:

- Sleep disorders
- Headache and migraine
- Heart irregularities
- Nausea
- Dizziness
- Rheumatic pain

and more

What is weather sensitivity?

Do you feel tired or exhausted? Do you suffer from headache? Why don't you blame the weather? Millions claim that the weather literally gets onto their nerves. Just because there is only limited scientific proof that weather sensitivity exists doesn't mean that you are wrong and doesn't mean that the medical profession should dismiss your plight as a psychological disorder. The sheer number of worldwide sufferers won't be ignored any longer—and science is slowly catching up.

Up to 60% of Germans claim to be weather sensitive but only 30% of Americans do, and hardly any citizens of other countries. Why the discrepancy? Critics say that people, rather than blaming their unhealthy lifestyle, search for something else to attribute their pain and suffering to. The media obliges and makes, in some countries more than others, the issue of 'weather and health' a hot topic. Others argue that the greater awareness of weather sensitivity in countries such as Germany and the US allows their citizens to speak out without fear of ridicule.

Whether we like it or not, you and I are part of nature. We are not robots but biological beings, evolved over millions of years. Despite technology's great efforts to detach us from nature, we are still subject to it, including the weather. Many animals and plants can sense changes in weather well in advance. Birds feel the drop in barometric pressure before the arrival of 'bad' weather and increase their foraging. Cats become restless, not only because they see Tweety foraging on the ground. Perhaps we have inherited some leftover weather sensitivity from our primeval ancestors as well.

A weather-sensitive person reacts with varying intensity to changes in weather elements, such as air pressure, temperature and humidity. These changes can affect a person's wellbeing and may worsen the symptoms of existing disorders, in particular pain. Some of the effects are:

- Increased irritability and aggressiveness, anxiety, depression, listlessness, fatigue, lack of concentration
- Sleep disorders
- Headache and migraine
- Heart and circulation irregularities
- Nausea
- Dizziness
- Scar pain or 'phantom pain'
- Rheumatic pain.

The symptoms vary from person to person and their intensity generally increases with age, lower level of fitness and a body weakened due to illness. Of course, they can also mask or be the result of an underlying disorder that has nothing to do with weather. Therefore, see your doctor if uncertain of the cause.

Patients who have had a heart attack are susceptible to weather sensitivity, sometimes extremely so. The rate is three times higher than it is in persons who never had a heart attack. Sensitivity persists for two to ten years after the attack. Scientists are now trying to find the weather situation that most influences these patients. Also, they are not sure whether the sensitivity is a result of the heart attack or the precursor to future problems.

'My grandfather's rheumatic knee hurts; we will get rain.' Many people trust their hips and knees and forecast the weather almost as accurately as can the meteorologists with their supercomputers. But why do some people respond to weather and others don't? Many theories abound, many surveys have been completed and much research conducted. But scientists agree to disagree.

Rapid and frequent weather changes appear to be the main culprits. Statistical evidence links increased numbers of many disorders and behaviour to certain weather conditions. Biometeorologists subdivided the passage of weather fronts into weather phases and compared the occurrence dates of each phase with hospital records. They found and published some startling relationships between weather and health. Critics could not dismiss the statistical evidence as pure coincidence.

> **Fight weather sensitivity**
>
> - Avoid overheated and stuffy rooms
> - Harden your senses by enjoying the outdoors in all weather conditions
> - Ensure regular sleep
> - Have a balanced and healthy diet
> - Treat sour moods with sunshine
> - Take alternating warm and cold showers
> - Participate in anti-stress therapies
>
> **Warning!** Symptoms of weather sensitivity may mask serious health problems. See your doctor if unsure.

Weather-sensitive people become irritated a day or two before the change and are often miserable when a weather front arrives. The conditions favour childbirth, so a greater number of babies have their first glimpses of their parents during those weather conditions. Cases of suicides, heart attacks, bleeding ulcers, headaches and migraines all increase. Rheumatics dread the arrival of cold and damp weather, while cold and dry air aggravates asthma symptoms. Expanding air in isolated body cavities may explain some weather-sensitivity symptoms. The weather fronts have something for everybody, it seems.

Some scientists take a different approach in their quest to solve the puzzle. They believe that electromagnetic impulses have an effect on our wellbeing. Natural electromagnetism, strong enough to cause weather sensitivity, is present in lightning-induced atmospherics (sferics) and charged particles (ions).

If weather can make you sick, it is no wonder that mood, performance and behaviour are also affected. Schoolchildren seem restless and distracted before a significant change in weather. Performance suffers and unruliness increases. Hey kids—now you can blame the weather!

Of course, the same goes for adults. In addition to increased irritability, aggressiveness and lack of concentration, your reaction times are slower during cloudy, hot and humid days that have falling barometric pressure and dry winds. Your reaction times are best during days of high pressure, sunshine and comfortable temperatures.

The passage of a cold front

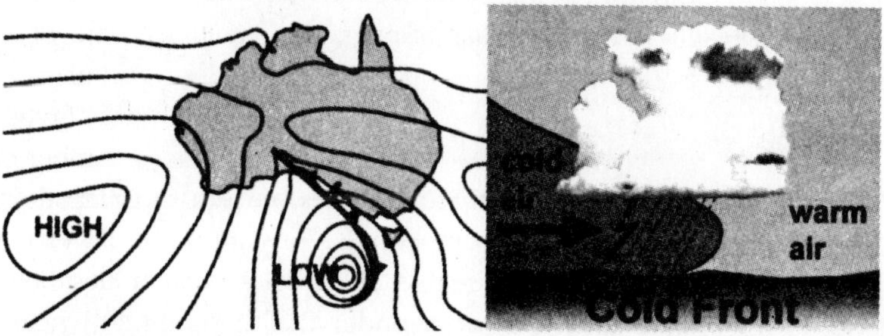

Situation: A front is about to cross SE Australia. Cold and humid maritime air wedges itself beneath warm and dry continental air, stirring up the atmosphere. Clouds thicken and showers and thunderstorms develop. The air pressure drops rapidly before the front arrives and rises equally as fast after the passage of the front. The temperature plummets and humidity rises. Strong and gusty winds shift from northwest to southwest.

Health: Weather-sensitive people become irritated and may develop headache/migraine before the front arrives. Cases of suicide, heart attack, bleeding ulcer, stroke, asthma attack, rheumatic pain, migraine and headache increase when the front passes. The situation also favours childbirth.

What can you do about weather sensitivity? It is likely that we all benefit from the frequent stimulation of changing weather. The modern lifestyle, with air conditioners, humidifiers and heaters, however, blunts the weather 'shocks'. In other words, we are no longer trained to cope with weather stress. Therefore, the best advice is to harden your senses by exposing them to the elements. Spend more time outdoors, in all kinds of weather. European medical professionals go even further and recommend stronger stimulants, such as saunas or alternating hot and cold showers.

Headache and migraine

When someone talks of weather sensitivity, the first thing that springs to mind is headache or migraine. The two conditions differ in their origin. Headache is the symptom of something else: substance abuse, tension, stress or an underlying medical condition. Migraine is a medical condition by itself and is the cause of migraine headache.

Headache

The hustle and bustle of modern life stretches our senses to the limits. Work becomes more and more competitive. Constant noise drowns out a 'quiet' moment. Add to it an excess of substances such as alcohol, nicotine or caffeine and it is no wonder that millions suffer from headache daily. It is one of the most common medical problems in today's world.

Everyone has a headache at one time or another: 'Not tonight darling, I've got a headache.' This is a phrase for so many jokes. But the pain of a headache is quite often incapacitating and nothing to laugh about. More than half the patients with tension-type headaches report moderate to severe impairments of their social and work activities. The number of people suffering from headache is unclear because aggressive advertising by pharmaceutical companies and easy access to over-the-counter drugs persuade many sufferers to treat themselves. The estimated occurrence in populations of developed countries ranges from 30% to 80%.

Headaches are often dismissed as trivial—after all, you can't die from headache. Yet they are the symptoms of a cause. Perhaps it is just your lifestyle, but the pain can also be a warning sign of more serious medical conditions.

There is a multitude of headache types. Some of these are:

- **Tension-type headache.** It is the most common type and mainly caused by stress, fatigue, depression and anxiety.
- **Sinus headache.** As the name suggests, sinus irritations or infections cause this headache.
- **Eyestrain headaches.** A modern type of headache due to long periods of concentrated focusing, such as computer work or reading.
- **Secondary headache.** This is the symptom of an underlying disorder.
- **Neuralgia.** Caused by irritated nerves.
- **Substance abuse headache.** Overindulgence in alcohol, nicotine, caffeine or other drugs often cause the 'hangover' effect.

Migraine

Migraine is more than a headache. It is a major symptom of a medical condition with strong and pulsating pain, generally on one side of the head. Nausea, vomiting, depression, and light and sound sensitivity quite often accompany the pain. A migraine attack can last for several hours or days and return periodically. An aura, either a visual disturbance or a feeling of numbness in the hands, arms and face, precedes a migraine attack in some patients.

For years, the medical profession has believed that blood flow changes in the brain are the cause of migraine headache. A trigger causes the blood vessels to constrict. As a consequence, the reduced blood flow carries less oxygen to the brain. The body reacts to this danger by widening the blood vessels again. The theory is that the swollen blood vessels pressure certain nerve fibres in the brain. In addition, several chemicals released during this process cause an inflammation and swelling of brain tissue and increase the sensitivity of pain receptors.

Updated imaging technology, however, has allowed researchers to study the blood flow changes during migraine attacks. They have found that these changes are much more complicated than the previous theory suggests. Many scientists now agree that migraine is a result of changes in the brain rather than the blood flow. This prompted others to suggest that migraine is an inherited disease.

Whatever the cause, we know the ailment affects millions of people all over the world. In Western countries, approximately 10 to 18% of the population suffer from migraine attacks. To put it more specifically, about 3 million Canadians and 26 million Americans complain of migraine, of which between 60 and 75% are women.

Weather Triggers

Weather features prominently as one of many environmental triggers of headache and migraine. A rapid change of single weather elements, such as barometric pressure, temperature, humidity or wind, and a combination of them in changing weather patterns are responsible for the onset of pain. Some scientists believe that a rapid change in weather—and possibly the ionization of the air—can alter the chemical balance in the human body.

Stress, however, is by far the most common trigger of headache and migraine. Surprisingly, weather changes run second and bright sunlight fourth. Headache and migraine sufferers implicate these weather conditions as either triggers or aggravating factors for their pain. Many studies and surveys confirm the 'imaginations' of sufferers. There is a relationship between weather factors and the onset of headache or migraine.

The complexity of interacting weather elements makes it hard for researchers to correlate pain with weather patterns. Nevertheless, an approaching weather front with falling air pressure, thickening clouds, rising humidity, temperature fluctuations and strengthening wind appear to trigger or aggravate more migraine attacks than any other weather pattern. In contrast, a dry day with high air pressure and sunshine soothes the symptoms.

Of course, there are always exceptions. For some people, a major trigger of headache and migraine is bright sunlight. Extremes in temperature and humidity appear to have a similarly negative effect on others.

Of all single weather elements, barometric pressure is the strongest factor. The barometric pressure can change significantly during the passing of a weather front. A rapid decrease and increase of 5% is not uncommon. The barometric pressure also fluctuates rapidly when winds buffet buildings.

Previously I mentioned the ability of birds to sense pressure changes. While scientists don't know exactly how they can, they do have a fair idea. The air inside a sealed cavity or sac, either in the ear or in the body, expands and contracts with the changes in barometric pressure—similar to the function of a barometer or altimeter. The senses of the birds are so finely tuned that they either detect the pressure changes within the cavity or they register the expansion of the sac.

Humans have plenty of cavities as well. Take the sinuses, for example. When the barometric pressure falls, the air inside the sinuses expands and any excess escapes via small openings into the nostrils. If the openings are blocked by mucus, as during a cold, then the pressure inside the sinuses builds up sufficiently to increase sinus pain and trigger a headache or migraine. Whether such changes in barometric pressure are enough to also affect blood vessels and fluid-filled cavities in the brain and inner ear, or whether they alter the chemical composition of the body, is under investigation. It is well documented, however, that some weather-sensitive people can 'feel' the arrival of a weather front many hours or a day in advance.

So-called ill winds also trigger headache and migraine amongst many people. The howling wind and the rattling of windows and shutters gets on your nerves. Warm, hot and very dry mountain and desert winds dry out the mucus membranes, irritate the airways and ionize the air. The populations of Alpine nations go crazy with headache and migraine when their *föhn* wind descends from the mountains, as do North Americans on *chinook* days, Israelis when the *sharav* blows and Australians on days with *easterlies, westerlies* or *northerlies*, depending on which part of the coast they live.

City life also causes headache, but its stress and noise aren't the only responsible factors. Add a little ozone, carbon monoxide and other chemicals to the atmosphere and the headache becomes a 'monster' headache. On warm and calm days, pollutants collect in the air and hang about the suburbs in stagnant clouds. The chemicals either trigger headache directly or, as is the case with carbon monoxide, reduce the amount of oxygen in the blood to cause headache indirectly. When the brain detects low levels of oxygen it initiates the widening of blood vessels to ensure supply. This dilation exerts pressure on parts of the brain and causes—you guessed it—headache. No wonder city people flock to the country to escape the stress and noise for some peace and quiet.

Studies suggest that environmental electromagnetism influences brain patterns, irritates nerves and changes body chemistry. Not so well researched is the possible negative effect of changes in the earth's electromagnetic field during solar storms on headache and migraine. More evidence is available, however, to support the theory of ionization as trigger. Ions are particles in the air with either too many negative electrons (negatively charged), or with missing electrons (positively charged). Positive ionization is said to cause the release of excessive serotonin into the bloodstream. The resulting constriction and dilation of blood vessels in the brain triggers the headache or migraine.

Weather triggers of headache and migraine

- Weather phases—falling air pressure, thickening clouds, rising humidity, temperature fluctuations and strengthening wind
- Rapid drops and rises in barometric pressure
- Dry and warm mountain and desert winds
- Stagnant and polluted air
- Extreme temperatures and humidity
- Bright sunlight
- Ionization of the atmosphere

Treatment

The aim of headache or migraine treatment is both to prevent and relieve or stop the painful symptoms. Headache and migraine are the most self-treated disorders. Painkillers, for adults and children, fly from the supermarket shelves like confectioneries. Many people seek medical advice only when the attacks become frequent or unbearable. Treating head pain with medication, however, is not a cure. You and your doctor need to find the source and the trigger of the symptoms.

Once it's identified, your doctor can target the source and recommend practices to avoid the triggers. Then prevention becomes as easy as avoiding the chocolate that provokes your migraine, or performing relaxation techniques to prevent your tension-type headache. Easier said then done—especially when weather is the trigger. To ascertain that weather is the trigger, keep a diary and note the type of weather factors that either bring about or increase your headache pain. Once identified, you can take preventative medication whenever this particular type of weather is forecast. Alternatively, follow the recommendations in the box 'Fight Weather Sensitivity' earlier in this chapter.

Rheumatism

'My joints ache.' This is a very general statement and doesn't give anyone a clue of the pain's cause. To call aching bones 'rheumatism' is also very general. Rheumatism is a collective word that refers to the pain of a variety of disorders, including inflamed, infected, injured or worn-out muscles and joints. Arthritis, a term often interchanged with rheumatism, is just one of its many ailments.

The following list includes three examples of common disorders:

- **Osteoarthritis** is one of the most common joint diseases. Wear and tear during someone's active life leaves them living their later years with painful and swollen joints. Sports injuries, repetitive strain, demanding physical labour and other factors often initiate the problems at an early age.
- **Rheumatoid arthritis** is not the result of wear and tear. Medical professionals believe it is an auto-immune disease, in which the body's immune system has gone awry and attacks itself. While it is mostly seen as disabling and destroying joints and surrounding tissue, rheumatoid arthritis sometimes attacks other body parts, such as the heart, lungs and eyes. Rheumatoid arthritis develops at any age, but most often between the ages of 20 and 50.
- **Fibromyalgia**, also known as muscular rheumatism or fibrositis, is an inflammation of muscle tissue. It causes pain and stiffness, particularly in the areas of neck, shoulders, hips and spine. The patient may also experience fatigue, sleep disorders and other symptoms. The disease can occur at any age.

Weather and Rheumatism

Research and surveys overwhelmingly support 'folklore' and anecdotal evidence of weather sensitivity amongst people with rheumatism. Some researchers go so far as building climate chambers where they can recreate certain weather conditions. Depending in which study and survey you want to believe, the proportion of people whose rheumatism was affected by weather ranges between 70% and 90%. One thing is clear, however: weather doesn't cause rheumatism and doesn't damage joints—but it does affect the severity of rheumatic pain.

Weather-sensitive people with rheumatism report more pain on damp, cold days that have rapidly falling barometric pressure. Thunderstorm activity and the ionization of the air can add to this. Depending on their type of rheumatic disorder, some people can predict well in advance the coming of a weather front, others 'feel' a nearby thunderstorm and some hear their joints tell them that it will rain. As with headache and migraine sufferers, the weather change takes the blame. But once the weather stabilizes the symptoms will, too.

Several theories exist on the mechanisms of weather sensitivity and rheumatism. One explains that the increased pain is due to the irritation of nerve ends from frequent and rapid changes in weather elements. Also, bones and muscles have different densities, and the unequal expansion and contraction during temperature and humidity variations may increase the pain in inflamed or injured joints and muscles.

Another plausible cause is the rapid change in barometric pressure before and during the passage of a weather front. Membranes and fluids in the joints expand when the outside barometric pressure drops. The expansion puts pressure on the inflamed tissue, causing increased pain. Some people with rheumatism also report increased pain during air travel in cabins with reduced air pressure.

Treatment

If cold and damp are the main culprits, why doesn't everyone with rheumatism move to warmer and drier climates? Some do, but recent evidence shows that pain due to changes in temperature and humidity is relative. Once your body acclimatizes to the warm and dry conditions, a drop of temperature and rise in humidity to levels that you found comfortable before the move causes almost the same negative symptoms. The perceived gain is so small that rheumatologists rarely recommend a change in location. Mind you, a 'friendlier' climate can have some emotional benefits—and a good mood makes pain more bearable.

Treatment with medication and physical therapy depends on the type of rheumatism. Doctors often recommend relaxation therapy and light exercises. Swimming, for instance, exercises the muscles without putting much strain on the joints. Anti-inflammatory drugs are the main weapons to combat the symptoms, while new drugs arrive on the market regularly. Complementary medicine, such as acupuncture and massage, can also provide some relief for sufferers.

Electromagnetic influences

Signor Luigi Galvani (1737–1798), an Italian anatomy professor, would today have a hard time explaining his experiments with animals. Inserting a copper hook into the spinal cord of a frog and hanging it on the balcony would surely whip up the passions of animal liberationists. The frog was presumably dead, let's hope, because the aim of the experiment was to bring it back to life—at least partially. In the manner of the fictional Dr. Frankenstein, he proved that the electrically charged air near a thunderstorm is enough to make a dead frog's leg twitch.

Researchers at the University of Giessen, Germany, had a similar idea in 1995. They tested 126 people for sensitivity to atmospheric electromagnetism, or *sferics.* No, they didn't use copper hooks and the subjects weren't exposed to lightning strikes. In a chamber that was gold plated to minimize outside interference, they simulated weak sferics similar to the naturally occurring variety near thunderstorms. The graphic record of the subjects' brain responses revealed heightened activity during the experiments. This brain activity was particularly high in a group of women known as being sensitive to weather.

If anything, this proves that to be human—to live—requires more than just water and chemical compounds. We need that proverbial 'spark' in our lives. Or to put it less dramatically, electronic impulses, together with chemical compounds, play a vital role in transmitting nerve and brain signals. Psychics tell us that they can feel or see a person's aura, the field of energy that surrounds every human being. Bio-Electrography, also known as Kirlian photography, named after a Russian scientist, reveals an energy corona around living objects on photographic paper or special video equipment.

You've probably heard that some animals, especially migratory birds, use an inbuilt 'compass' and the earth's magnetic field to navigate. Scientists have found a magnetic mineral called magnetite in the brain tissue which acts as the sensor. Zoologists currently discuss the possibility that some whales use the same technique. Disturbances in the magnetic field would, therefore, explain whale beachings.

In 1979, students of the University of Manchester, England, became the 'pigeons' in a test to search for leftover homing capabilities in humans. The blindfolded students were driven for an hour on winding roads and then asked to point into the direction of their campus. Most were fairly accurate.

The test could be pure coincidence, but today we know that the human brain contains magnetite as well. The challenge is to find out the amount and what the mineral is doing in our brains in the first place. Since you and I are living on a giant magnet, the earth, some form of interference with our nervous system is the logical consequence. Magnetite in the brain could at least explain the ability of some people to 'feel' the charged atmosphere of an approaching thunderstorm.

You and I are constantly exposed to the electromagnetic radiation from microwave ovens, radio and television sets, computer terminals, power lines, mobile phones and a growing list of other sources. You read stories of greater numbers of cancer victims who lived near power lines and of the possible risk of 'frying' your brain when using a mobile phone. The WHO wants to put matters to rest and is funding a project to study the health effects of electromagnetic fields (EMFs).

If the doomsayers are right, hopefully we can do something about man-made magnetism in the future. There is not much we can do, however, against the wide range of natural electromagnetism. Two types are strong enough to grab the attention of biometeorologists: atmospheric discharges (sferics), and the ionization of the atmosphere (ions).

Sferics

Sferics is short for atmospherics, the name radio operators gave to the crackling noise in their loudspeakers and headphones, caused by nearby or distant lightning. The US Lightning Detection Network registers over

20 million lightning flashes per year, while worldwide the estimate is 100 strikes per second. In addition, many discharges occur high in the atmosphere and remain undetected.

A multimillion-volt lightning bolt announces its presence by sending out electromagnetic signals, sferics, with the speed of light. They are strong enough to twitch nearby dead frog legs, as in Signor Galvani's experiment, and to sour milk. Further away—instruments can measure them hundreds of kilometres away—cats get nervous and ants prepare their mounds in preparation for the expected rain and wind. Some scientist believe that sferics are also the main cause of weather sensitivity in humans.

Headaches are the main symptoms of this kind of weather sensitivity. But statistical evidence also implicates sferics with emotional stress and mood swings, irregularities with heart rhythm and blood circulation, and epileptic attacks.

Ions

Right now you are breathing electricity. I am too, and everybody else. All the atoms, molecules and airborne particles are home to electrons. Electrons are negatively charged and provide a balance to the positive centre of the particle. When a particle loses a negative electron, the positive force is stronger—the particle becomes a *positive ion*. The lost electron is likely to attach to a different particle. This can cause an over-population of negative electrons and create a *negative ion*. The air is *ionized* when large quantities of either type of ion exist.

Nature forces the migration of electrons in several ways. For example, X-rays and UV radiation split electrons from their host. Collisions and friction amongst particles, caused by air turbulence or water movement, also ionizes the air. The negative ions near waterfalls, ocean waves and amongst the rustling leaves in forests may have something to do with the calming effect of these environments on people. On the other hand, positive ions in polluted air and near synthetic building materials and clothing are thought to be detrimental to a person's wellbeing. Advocates of this theory recommend the use of negative ion generators.

Critics argue that ions don't live very long. This is true. They prefer to be *neutral* and pass on the excess electron to needy neighbours. Independent ions don't live longer than five minutes, while clumps of ions survive for up to 20 minutes. Nevertheless, as long as the cause of the ionization exists, the supply won't run out.

The quantity of ions in the air depends largely on the weather conditions. In dry conditions, ions tend to survive longer and are, therefore, in greater numbers. Certain mountain and desert winds contain large quantities of positive ions. People exposed to these winds often display initial euphoria followed by headache, migraine, depression or exhaustion. Lightning is a major producer of either type of ions. Humid and foggy conditions reduce the numbers.

Research into the effect of ions on human health is very inconsistent. Some research papers provide undeniable proof while others conclude the opposite. Perhaps, as is the case with sferics, individuals react differently to ion exposure, or not at all. Some evidence points to benefits in treating respiratory problems, such as asthma, bronchitis and hay fever, with ionized air. The theory is that ions act on the nerve fibres in the airways, and influence the production of mucus and the movement of the cilia, the tiny hair-like organs that clean the airways.

Ill winds

Police car sirens whine through city streets. Officers are busy attending unusually high numbers of car accidents, rowdy crowd behaviour, domestic violence and suicides. Hospitals overflow and the undertakers count the cash. Long-term residents know what is driving everybody crazy—the hot and dry wind that is blowing down the mountain range or out of arid regions. They call it the *föhn* in Central Europe, *chinook* and *Santa Ana* in North America, *sharav* in Israel, and a *northerly, westerly* or *easterly* in Australia. Every country has its own name for the ill winds.

What makes these winds so unbearable? Meteorologists and medical scientists of Alpine countries studied these winds for many years and confirmed a link between increases in accident, crime and suicide rates and the onset of the *föhn*. The *chinook* in the Rocky Mountains takes the blame for migraine and the *sharav* in Israel is said to cause weather sensitivity.

While there is enough statistical evidence to prove a relationship between the ill winds and wellbeing, scientists concentrate their research

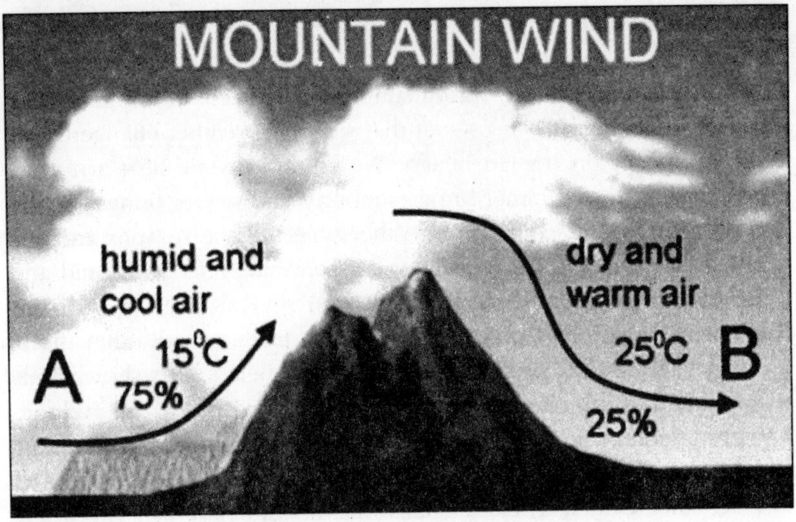

on specific elements of the winds. It is most likely a combination of all the following four factors:

1 The winds are generally very dry. A mountain wind loses most of its moisture in the rain on the mountain's side facing the wind, while the humidity in desert winds can be almost non-existent. The air dries the mucus membranes in the airways and sinuses. Then airborne germs, dust and pollen can easily get past the dry mucus and cause inflammation, irritation or an allergic reaction. The dry winds may also trigger asthma, migraine and sinusitis-related headache.
2 The temperature rises with the onset of the winds. In winter, springtime temperatures arrive within a few hours and in summer the mercury reaches heat wave levels. The short-term rises in temperature may cause springtime lethargy and other heat-related body reactions, such as rashes and cramps.
3 The winds are strong and often blow for weeks, sometimes months—enough to get on anyone's nerves. Buffeting by winds causes rapid fluctuations in air pressure, thus triggering weather sensitivity.
4 The friction between the land's surface and the wind dislodges electrons from airborne particles, so that the mountain and desert winds contain a high proportion of positive ions. Respiratory problems, headache, depression and exhaustion are linked to positive ions.

Seasonal health

The first warm rays of the spring sun magically seem to improve your sense of wellbeing. It is no secret that seasonal weather changes have a strong impact on human health. We know extreme heat and cold makes us sick, that summer brings sunburns and winter brings coughs and sneezes. Scientists delved into the subject of the seasons and our health a little deeper, and found some astonishing relationships.

Researchers correlated death rates from several diseases with the dates of the death and observed the trend. Infectious diseases, heart problems and strokes peak in winter. Extreme heat events show short-term peaks in death rates from heart-related disorders. On the average, however, winter cold appears to increase the rate of death from almost all diseases. A noticeable exception is cancer, which is equally spread amongst the seasons. The seasonal variability of death rates is greatest amongst the elderly above 60 years of age. Also, men appear to be more susceptible to cold influences, while women succumb to heat extremes more often.

There are regional differences, though. In climates with few dramatic temperature changes, death rates from infectious diseases showed most seasonal fluctuations. Changes in local weather conditions, such as the onset of the wet or dry season in the tropics, impact on the numbers of disease carriers and the survivability of viruses ,and bacteria.

Researchers took a further step and correlated birthdays with birth rates. Surprise! They observed marked seasonal variations. The birth of animals almost always follows the seasons. But in their case, the availability of food dictates evolution. Human reproduction appears to follow some other rules. For example, statistics show a lowering of the conception rate by 6 to 10% after a period with temperatures of up to 10 degrees above average. A low sperm count is to blame. This should reflect in less births during spring, and it does. Whether the fertility of women is also influenced by seasonal weather changes is unclear.

The birth rate may be lower, but springtime produces the heaviest and largest newborns. Babies born in spring are taller and heavier than those born during other months. Danish mothers, giving birth in this season, find their bundle to be an average 2.2 mm longer than those ffom mothers giving birth in winter. Eighteen-year-old Austrian soldiers with springtime birthdays are on average 6 mm taller than their companions born in autumn. Austrian researchers speculate that a difference in sunshine hours during pregnancy is a factor.

Seasonal factors also appear to affect the fetal and infant mortality rates, and the numbers of babies born with defects. Infant mortality peaks during summer heat-stress periods. More infants with diabetes are born during spring and early summer; and more schizophrenia appears amongst babies born in late winter and spring. Infectious diseases during the winter months, the seasonality of hormone changes, and nutritional or environmental factors, are all possible causes.

Winter is the season of colds, influenza and respiratory diseases. No secret here? Yes, there is. Like humans, bacteria and viruses prefer a warm climate. So why do they cause widespread outbreaks during winter? The winter months are generally more humid and have less UV radiation. Germs love the moisture and hate the sterilizing effect of the sun's radiation. We also tend to spend more time indoors where the germs can accumulate. In addition, low temperatures in winter stress the immune system. Invaders encounter weakened defences.

A season with warm and humid weather breeds disease carriers such as the mosquito. In the tropics, the wet season is host to a variety of infectious diseases. Warm and dirty drinking water is also a breeding ground for viruses and bacteria. Hot summers in temperate regions often signal outbreaks of food poisoning. Poor food storage and handling techniques can leads to a rapid growth of bacteria numbers.

Chapter Three

Air

Blame the air for:

- Heart disorders
- Bronchitis
- Hay fever
- Asthma
- Infectious diseases

  and more

Something in the air

Air is a reservoir of breathable gases. Air is the window that shields life from deadly radiation. Air is the earth's armour that protects against meteorite bombardments. Air is a blanket that keeps the earth warm. Air is the carrier of energy and water. Air is a garbage disposal system.

The six sentences above briefly describe the main functions of air rather than define what it is. Without air, the earth would be a lifeless, rock-strewn planet. So, what is this air you breathe?

Clean and dry air, that is, air without water vapour and airborne substances, is a mixture of several gases. Nitrogen (78%), oxygen (21%) and argon (0.9%) are the main constituents. The leftover space (0.1%) is reserved for carbon dioxide, methane, neon, helium, krypton, hydrogen,

Composition of the atmosphere below 25 km

Component	Symbol	Volume % (dry air)
Nitrogen	N_2	78.08
Oxygen	O_2	20.98
Argon	Ar	0.93
Neon	Ne	0.0018
Helium	He	0.0005
Hydrogen	H_2	0.00005
Krypton	Kr	0.0011
Xenon	Xe	0.00009
Carbon dioxide	CO_2	Variable
Ozone	O_3	Variable
Methane	CH_4	Variable
Sulphur dioxide	SO_2	Variable
Water vapour	H_2O	Maximum 4%

xenon, and ozone. All these gases generally mingle well amongst each other. The exception is ozone. It concentrates in the ozone layer (stratospheric ozone)—at an altitude about 10–50 km high in the atmosphere—and may be present near the earth's surface (ground-level ozone).

The air is hardly ever dry, though, as almost three quarters of the earth's surface beneath it is water. Some of this water evaporates and forms an invisible, odourless gas—water vapour. The earth's solid crust, its plants and animals and sweaty humans, also pass some moisture to the atmosphere. The amount of water vapour in the atmosphere determines humidity.

Water vapour doesn't replace the other gases of the air completely. The maximum volume that is available is 4%. Once this amount is reached, the air is saturated and the water vapour has filled all available space (100% relative humidity).

Excess water vapour condenses and forms tiny water droplets in the air. At sufficiently low temperatures, the droplets freeze into small ice crystals. The suspended droplets and ice crystals appear as clouds, fog or mist.

The constituents of the air are dense enough to form a protective barrier against most cosmic meteorites and radiation. The friction of the air burns up small and fast-moving intruders, but large meteorites occasionally reach the ground and cause damage. The air also absorbs most of the sun's harmful radiation, although obviously enough heat energy reaches the surface to sustain life.

The earth loses approximately as much heat energy as it gains. Clouds and features on the surface reflect some of the incoming rays. The surface itself radiates heat back into space, particularly at night. But clouds act as a blanket and keep some of the radiation at home. A cloudy night is, therefore, warmer than a clear night. Also, various gases and man-made pollutants upset the energy balance. They trap heat energy and cause a steady climb of the earth's average temperature (global warming).

With so many ingredients in it, the air has to weigh something—and it does. While a bag full of air doesn't weigh much, all the air above you is quite heavy. A column of 1 cm^2 extending into space weighs about 1 kg. Depending on the size of your shoulders, they have to bear more than 500 kg of air. This weight, however, is not only exerted downwards but sideways and upwards as well. In other words, it creates pressure in all directions. The air pressure inside your body equals that of the outside, thus preventing you from being squashed.

Atmosphere

Like the skin of an apple that tightly surrounds the fleshy interior, the air also hugs close to the surface of the earth. Almost all air resides within 80 km of height. Compare this with the earth's diameter of 12,756 km and the comparison to an apple's thin skin is well justified. The ancient Greeks called this skin *atmos sphaira* (vapour ball); today we call it atmosphere. Because air is highly compressible, its own weight squeezes about 50% of its content to within the first 5 km of height. Mountain climbers who venture above this height have to carry compressed air. Aircraft compensate for the lack of air by pressurizing cabins.

In addition to a decreasing air pressure with height, other elements also undergo changes. The temperature, for example, decreases at certain heights and increases at others. It is, therefore, quite logical that scientists divided the atmosphere into layers according to their temperature characteristics. They named five layers:

- **Troposphere.** The troposphere, the layer immediately above the earth's surface, contains almost all water vapour and weather occurrences. The top of the troposphere, the tropopause, varies between 8 km over the poles and 16 km over the equator. The temperature decreases with height and drops to –50°C over the poles and –90°C over the equator.

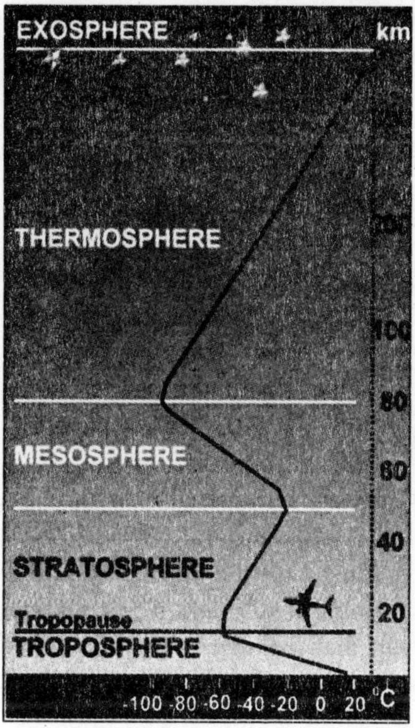

- **Stratosphere.** Where the temperature stops decreasing, the stratosphere begins. This reversal in temperature lapse, an inversion, prevents vertical air movements. Airline passengers enjoy a smooth flight in the lower parts of the stratosphere. The stratosphere is home to the ozone layer.
- **Mesosphere.** Between 50 and 80 km above us lies the mesosphere. It is characterized by another drop in temperature; to as low as –90°C.
- **Thermosphere.** The thin air of the thermosphere lets the sun's radiation enter the layer almost unhindered. Anything within the thermosphere, including the air's molecules, heat up very quickly during the day and temperatures can reach extremes of 600°C—much more during solar storms.
- **Exosphere.** Above 500 km extends the suitably named exosphere—the exit to space. The air is so thin that satellites can orbit without much resistance.

Pollution

Unfortunately, the air is never pure. Many natural and man-made impurities, called aerosols, are adrift. Suspended particles of a natural origin are sea salt, sand, organic dust, pollen and smoke. Millions of years ago, the natural pollutants of volcanoes and the dust from meteor strikes were enough to poison the air and change the earth's climate, altering much of life on earth. Many species perished, while others evolved. Today, however, it is the man-made pollution that is of great concern.

> **Smog Alert, London, 1991**
>
> For almost four days in December 1991, London experienced its worst smog since 1952. Nitrogen dioxide levels reached levels four times higher than the recommended maximum set by the WHO. An extra 160 people are thought to have died from respiratory and cardiovascular diseases

The unprecedented population explosion of the modern age brought with it the need for energy. Almost all this energy required around the world is still created by burning fossil fuels. The resulting industry and transport create pollution that makes air in some areas unhealthy. As a consequence, affected people suffer from diseases and die prematurely. Pollution damages agricultural crops, destroys historical monuments, and changes the climate. Relevant terms, such as 'acid rain', 'smog alert', 'global warming' and 'greenhouse effect', are common today.

National and international legislation resulted in a reduction of certain pollutants. Since the ban of lead as an additive to automotive fuel, it is no longer a major concern in most cities. Countries agreed to phase out the 'greenhouse' gases chlorofluorocarbon (CFC) and halon, but other damaging gases are still increasing in volume, especially in developing countries.

As an interim measure, or perhaps as a token gesture, health authorities issue smog alerts and air-quality warnings to the public. While you can't stop breathing the filthy air, if you do have lung or heart problems, you can consider precautionary measures, such as the avoidance of strenuous exercise. Some cities experience levels of pollution that even require emergency action plans.

Australian Air Quality Index		US Air Quality Index		Hong Kong Air Quality Index	
Air quality	Index	Descriptor	Index	Pollution level	Index
Very Good	0–33	Good	0–50	Low	0–5
Good	34–66			Medium	26–0
Fair	67–99	Moderate	51–100	High	51–00
Poor	100–149	Unhealthy for Sensitive Groups	101–150	Very High	101–00
Very Poor	150+	Unhealthy	151–200		
		Very Unhealthy	201–300	Severe	200+
		Hazardous	301–500		

Governments have set certain standards for each pollutant: nitrogen dioxide, sulphur dioxide, ozone, carbon monoxide and particulate matter (small suspended particles). They form the basis for an Air Quality Index (AQI). The standards, however, vary around the world, as does the index.

Weather and pollution

The weather can again be held accountable for the fact that pollution has become an international problem. Wind carries the waste of an industrial region to otherwise pristine regions. Fish die in Swedish lakes as a result of pollutants from Central Europe. Similarly, remote Canadian regions suffer from polluted air created in US industries hundreds of kilometres away. One estimate claims that 50% of sulphate deposits in Canada come from its southern neighbour. Ironically, the complaints of residents near industrial sites led to taller smokestacks that distribute the pollutants over a much larger area, letting neighbouring provinces suffer for a while.

For years, scientists believed that pollution would dilute into the atmosphere to negligible levels. Recent studies, however, showed otherwise. Certain wind patterns can carry the pollutants as a 'parcel' and deliver it many hundreds of kilometres away. At its destination, it may arrive as acid rain or snow over a limited area. Even the Arctic isn't spared. Mercury concentrations in Arctic spring rain or snow have more than tripled over the last two centuries.

Pollutants undergo some chemical changes while in the atmosphere and can reside there for a long time. Vertical mixing, i.e. updraughts and downdraughts, distribute the pollutants within the whole troposphere. Therefore, a European or Australian chemical can catch a ride in the global wind pattern and contribute to international pollution problems.

Strong winds and vertical mixing are also to blame for natural pollutants—dust and sand. For citizens at the edge of deserts, dust storms and sandstorms are a regular occurrence. Sahara dust and sand sometimes rise up to 5 km into the atmosphere and drift across the Atlantic. Several hundred million tons of dust leave the West African coast annually. The heavy particles settle in the Atlantic but lighter dust creates haze in the Caribbean, and meteorological authorities need to declare pollution alerts.

What does nice weather mean to you: light wind, no rain and glorious sunshine? Millions, however, relate nice weather with smog alerts and high pollution levels. In light or no wind conditions, the pollutants remain at home. Without vertical mixing, they accumulate and can exceed acceptable levels. If this is not enough, sunshine converts chemicals such as nitrogen dioxide into toxic ozone. So much for nice weather.

A stable atmosphere—one without updraughts—occurs frequently in winter during high-pressure situations. Instead of rising, the air actually descends and traps pollutants. A high-pressure system generally covers a large area and often remains active for many days, sometimes weeks. Thus, pollution gradually spreads over hundreds of kilometres.

When air descends it also warms. This can create a relatively warm layer of air above the cooler air near the surface—a temperature inversion. Warm polluted air from a smoke stack or car exhaust rises as long as it is warmer than the cooler surrounding air. When it reaches the warm layer it may have the same temperature and stops its rise. Instead, it spreads below the temperature inversion.

Inversions are the worst weather situation for the populations of major cities. Once enough particles have assembled, a thick layer of haze forms over the region. With even the slightest horizontal movement of the air, the haze spreads over large areas. But many cities are in valleys that prevent the gentle horizontal movement of the air, leading to a rapid increase in pollution levels, and authorities end up issuing a smog alert.

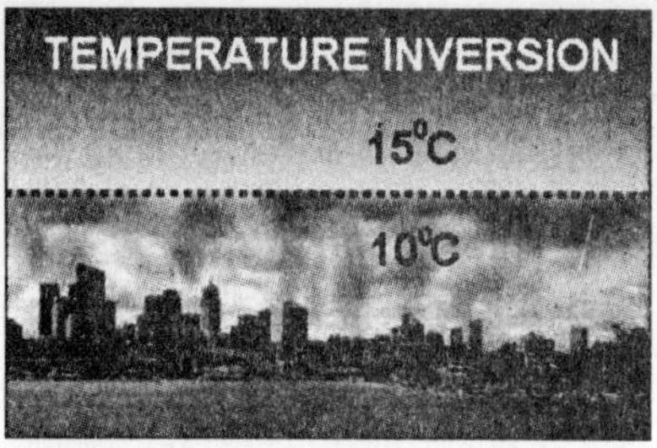

The term 'smog' first described a mixture of fog and smoke. Today it is also used to simply characterize heavily polluted air. In smog, pollutants reach such a high concentration that they exceed the standards. The mixture of industrial gases, vehicle exhausts and airborne particles in smog are harmful to all humans, regardless of their health status.

AIR AND HEALTH

Polluted air

Global air circulation ensures that long-life pollutants spread to all parts of the world. They pose a threat to us when their numbers overwhelm the self-cleaning ability of our respiratory system, or our immune system can't defend against the intruders.

Breathing isn't the only way that we are exposed to airborne pollutants and disease-causing microbes. These substances are continually deposited in the soil as dry fallout or precipitation. From the soil they enter the food chain and, ultimately, your body. Overall, your body absorbs more of a particular chemical via intake of food than through breathing. But some harmful substances only exist in gaseous form, and others, such as particulate matter, are only a health risk while airborne.

There is no doubt that airborne impurities bring illness and death. Air pollution disasters, such as London's 'killer smog' in 1952 that killed about 4,000 people, are thankfully rare today. Nevertheless, the ill effects are still with us (see table on p. 38) and even just a few hundred deaths are too many.

Estimated health impact of ambient air pollution in Europe

Health deficiency	Estimated number of cases (annual)
Cough and eye irritation in children	2.6–4 million
Lower respiratory illness in children	4–6 million
Lower respiratory illness in children causing a medical visit	17–29 thousand
Ambulatory visits due to respiratory disease	90–200 thousand
Decrease of pulmonary function by more than 5%	14 million
Incidence of chronic obstructive pulmonary disease	18–42 thousand
Hospital admissions due to respiratory disease	4–8 thousand

WHO European Centre for Environment and Health

The body is like a storage cabinet for toxic substances. A drawer may contain lead or mercury, while another may store modern chemical compounds, such as dioxins or pesticides. Each individual substance accumulates over the years until the drawer is full and eventually overcomes the body's tolerance. Yet research suggests that an interaction of even low levels of several chemicals can produce Multiple Chemical Sensitivity (MCS).

Chemicals suspended in the air also interact and form new substances. A typical example is the formation of acid particles and ozone. The strong irritant sulphur dioxide can, in combination with water droplets, form damaging acid. Medical examinations of children living in areas with high acid particle concentrations showed above-average numbers of bronchitis cases, and more children with restricted lung functions.

Bright sunlight converts nitrogen dioxide and volatile organic compounds to harmful ground-level ozone. Ozone attacks the mucus membranes of the airways, causing wheezing, coughing and infections. Exposure to high levels of ozone can lead to the development of asthma. Data from several studies also link ozone to an increased death rate amongst vulnerable persons.

Heavily polluted air is a health risk for everyone. At particular risk are:

- **People who exert themselves** during episodes of high pollution levels. Outdoor workers, athletes and people participating in strenuous outdoor activities breathe fast and deep to supply the body with additional oxygen. Along with the oxygen, however, more pollutants reach the lungs. Because some pollutants, in particular ozone, can impair the lung function, the muscles don't receive the required oxygen and so underperform.
- **Infants and children** are more likely to suffer from polluted air than healthy adults. Relative to their body size, children breathe a high volume of air, and breathe quickly. In addition, their underdeveloped respiratory system easily becomes irritated. The most recent studies also found a link between air pollution and an impaired immune system in children.
- **People already suffering from existing respiratory disorders** often have their symptoms of asthma, bronchitis, emphysema and other lung diseases intensified due to air pollutants.

Dry air

Some mountain and desert winds (*föhn, chinook, Santa Ana, sharav,* etc.) are very dry. Towns at the edge of arid areas experience seasonal winds with almost no moisture in the air, and many days and weeks with relative humidity levels below 10%. Your skin is dry; not a pearl of sweat in sight. Your perspiration evaporates without you noticing it. Dehydration is a real danger at such times.

Besides dehydration, dry air also promotes cracked skin and lips, and the drying of the mucus in your airways and sinuses. The sticky substance in your nose becomes hard as diamonds, and if you can't resist the urge to pick at it, it may result in bleeding. Bacteria and viruses don't like the dry conditions, but surviving germs find your dry and inflamed nose rather inviting and can get easily past the dried-up defence mechanism. In any case, with the entrance to your sinuses sometimes blocked, excess mucus can't drain, resulting in sinus problems.

The next time you get zapped by static electricity when exiting your car or touching a door handle, remember this explanation: the air is most likely very dry, so doesn't conduct well and static electricity builds up in your body to be discharged to a better conductor. The electric charge may act on your nervous system and cause irritation.

Odour

Do you live near a tannery or piggery, or does the smell of the local waste disposal site drift across your home? If so, then you'd know that unwelcome odour can be more than a nuisance. Odour is not a health hazard and is very subjective. But it can certainly bring about a foul mood. How can you blame the weather for a bad smell? Odour is a gas produced by chemicals or bacteria. Microbes love warm weather, multiply fast and produce a lot of gas while digesting whatever they are eating. It takes a little wind from a certain direction to blow the smell into your backyard.

Piggery waste turned to odourless fertiliser

A pig farmer has found a way of converting piggery waste into organic fertiliser that has no smell.

It has taken three years and $750,000 for Rob Brooks to develop the plant at Tansey in the Kilkivan shire, along with a Federal innovation grant of $189,000.

The project is expected to create up to six jobs.

Mr Brooks says the project has export potential, but the initial plan is to satisfy the domestic market needs.

'A lot of piggeries are in the same position as my own, whereby we have to do something with the solid waste,' he said.

'We're hoping that through this new plant, we will be able to use their waste product, pay them a price which is attractive for it, and everybody will be a winner out of it.'

ABC News Online, 9 January 2001

Main types of pollutants

Pollutant	Source	Major health effects
Carbon monoxide	Car exhausts, incomplete burning of fossil fuels	Replaces oxygen in the blood. Causes fatigue, dizziness, nausea, vomiting and headaches.
Sulphur dioxide	Processing and burning of fossil fuels in automobiles, industry and homes.	Irritates throat, lung and eyes. Narrows the airways, causing coughs and wheezes.
Nitrogen dioxide	Burning of fossil fuels in automobiles, industry and homes	Irritates throat, lung and eyes. Increased risk of developing respiratory infections.
Ozone	Nitrogen oxides react in sunlight with volatile organic compounds (photochemical reaction)	Irritates throat, lung and eyes. Narrows the airways, causing coughs and wheezes.
Lead	Exhaust gases from motor vehicles that use leaded petrol	Affects the nervous system, the body's ability to make blood and the mental development of children.
Volatile Organic Compounds (VOCs)	Industrial processes, evaporation of fuels and solvents.	Irritate the throat, lungs and eyes. Some cause headache and nausea, damage the liver, kidneys and nervous system, or are carcinogenic.
Particulate matter	Industrial and natural smoke. Soil, sand, dust and sea spray.	Irritates throat, lung and eyes. May cause and aggravate respiratory diseases. Associated with heart and circulatory disorders.

Respiratory disorders

When a film director tries to simulate a lack of oxygen in an aircraft cabin or a mining shaft, he asks the actors to desperately gulp for air and die very dramatically. The reality is different, however: you can breathe air without oxygen and not even realize that you will slowly fall asleep and die. A person only panics when the airflow is blocked or not enough air is available.

It is the oxygen that our lungs are after. About 300 million tiny air sacs in the lung, the alveoli, help the blood absorb the oxygen and dispose of the waste, carbon dioxide. An adult recycles about 10 litres of air per minute. A small child, relative to its body weight, breathes approximately three times as much. An exercising adult can exchange up to 50 litres per minute. Without a self-cleansing process, the sacs would fill very quickly with air impurities. The hair and the mucus lining in your nose should catch bacteria, dust and other intruders. But if the invader manages to sneak past, the cilia, small hair-like organs in the airways, move in a wave-like motion to convey it back to the outside. If this is not enough, you can also cough or sneeze to dislodge the foreign objects.

Heavily polluted air, however, can overwhelm the self-cleansing process, irritate the mucous membranes, or inhibit the movement of the cilia. Gases, such as ozone, bypass the self-defence mechanisms and reach the alveoli unhindered. Ozone is known to irritate and inflame the airways and possibly damages cells. Recent studies even implicate ozone with damage to the DNA.

Medical scientists are also concerned about the impact that fine airborne particles (particulate matter) has on human health. Only recently they discovered that microscopic aerosols, solid and liquid, penetrate deep into lung tissue where they can become permanently lodged. Studies of children, living in areas with air pollution, clearly associate fine particles with coughing, wheezing and bronchitis.

This shouldn't be a surprise. City air contains up to 100 billion particles per cubic metre. But even low concentrations can trigger significant symptoms of respiratory problems. As a result, health authorities of many countries revised their national standards for particulate matter concentrations.

Heart disorders

The number of hospital admissions of patients with cardiovascular disorders increases sharply on days with high concentrations of ozone and particulate matter. In some patients with underlying heart diseases, particulate matter alters the heart rate significantly enough to cause an attack.

The studies are new and incomplete. So far, they could not prove a link between pollution and the onset of cardiovascular problems in healthy people. It is known, however, that every major urban centre has ozone and particulate concentration levels high enough to pose a health risk several times per year. There is enough circumstantial evidence to suggest that pollution together, with other factors, can be enough to stress the heart of healthy people as well.

Bronchitis

Bronchitis is an inflammation or irritation of the linings of the airways (bronchial tubes). The inflamed tubes swell and produce a thick layer of mucus. This restricts the airflow, makes breathing difficult and is often accompanied by a whistling sound, or wheezing. Sometimes breathing is painful and the afflicted person will feel a tightness in their chest. The body reacts by forcing the sufferer to cough out some of the mucus.

There are two types of bronchitis: acute and chronic. Acute bronchitis is a short-term disorder. In most cases a viral infection is the cause, similar to that of the common cold and also contagious. Environmental factors are more often to blame for the longer-lasting chronic bronchitis. The ailment may plague a person for several months and even years. Smoking cigarettes is the main cause of chronic bronchitis, but long-term exposure to pollutants is also becoming a common cause. The airways have to produce additional mucus to combat the foreign substances. Coughing dislodges some of the mucus and propels it into the outside world—not a pretty sight. Coughing continues as long as the irritant is present, and the lungs are more susceptible to infection.

Because chronic bronchitis is the result of long-term exposure to irritants, it affects more people over 45. Of course, people at very high risk of developing bronchitis are smokers and those exposed to high concentrations of dust and fumes in their work environment. The slow advance of the disease makes it dangerous. People get used to the coming and going of the coughs and wheezes, and it becomes a fact of life. They may not realize for a long time that the symptoms occur more often and intensify. By the time they see a health professional, the lungs are seriously damaged. Lung diseases are the fourth leading cause of death in the United States.

The removal of the cause is the common treatment. As long as the irritant is present in the air the disease will continue. The patient must avoid polluted air and give up smoking. Medication can make some symptoms more bearable. Antibiotics reduce the impact of infections and bronchodilators open the airways.

Hay fever

For many people, the advent of the warm season is nothing to cheer about. Clouds of tree and grass pollen make their eyes water as if they were dicing onions and their wastepaper baskets overflow with tissues. An estimated 10–20% of the population do indeed find that spring can really hang you up the most, as they suffer from seasonal allergic rhinitis, better known as hay fever.

Hay fever is a form of allergic rhinitis. But, while allergic rhinitis is an almost constant reaction to a particular substance (allergen), hay fever comes and goes with the seasons: the flowering seasons of trees and grasses, and the sporing seasons of fungi.

Hay fever has become epidemic with modern times. Every year, medical practitioners of many countries report an increase in consultation numbers. A better awareness amongst the population and/or an increased willingness to consult a professional explains the rising numbers.

The symptoms of hay fever are similar to those of the common cold. The intensity, however, varies greatly between individuals. For some it is just a minor nuisance, while others find their daily activities disrupted. In severe cases, the patient develops asthma.

The main symptoms are:

- Congested or runny nose
- Frequent sneezing
- Watery or itchy eyes
- Itchy throat, nose or ear
- Wheezing and coughing
- Headache caused by blocked sinuses.

Pollen from trees, grasses and weeds are the most common triggers of allergic reactions. Less common, but also important, are the spores of a large variety of fungi. Generally, spring and summer are the worst seasons for sufferers. Some weeds and grasses, however, mature late in autumn. Autumn is also the season when the farmers cut grass to make hay. Haymaking not only releases pollen and fungus spores, but is also a very dusty business.

Air pollution will aggravate the irritation and swelling of airways. Studies show that pollution increases the sensitivity to allergens. Sufferers of rhinitis become more responsive to allergens when exposed to high doses of ozone, while a link has been established between an increased sensitivity to pollen and vehicle exhaust pollutants, in particular diesel fumes. As a result, the numbers of patients with hay fever are greater in cities than they are in rural areas.

To make matters worse, pollen cells rupture during and after rain and in periods of lightning. The pollen grains literally explode and release allergen-containing granules. Air samples taken in Australia after a bout of rain contained up to 50 times more allergens than in equivalent samples taken on a dry day.

When an allergen attaches itself to the surface of the airways or the eyes, the immune system of sensitive people mistakes the harmless intruder for a dangerous substance and overreacts. Cells can break down and release histamine, a chemical compound that causes swelling, itching and increased mucus flow or tears.

Hay fever is sometimes hereditary. The mechanisms behind this type, however, aren't completely understood at this stage. Some research suggests that children of parents with allergies become susceptible later in life. Also, some evidence exists that exposure to allergens as an infant increases the likelihood of developing an allergy as an adult.

Because pollen and spores float easily in the air, updraughts and wind play a vital role in distributing the particles. The first warm days in spring produce vertical air currents, called thermals, that carry the allergens high into the atmosphere. There they catch a ride in the prevailing winds and travel several hundred kilometres before they settle down. Therefore, you can't necessarily blame your neighbour's flowering ragweed for your stuffy nose.

If the pollen and spores miss the ride, they will settle nearby when the air cools in the evening. Cool and humid air for most of the day will discourage them to travel in the first place. As mentioned earlier, rain can increase the pollen concentration in the short term. But rain is welcomed by hay fever sufferers, nevertheless, as the allergens eventually wash away.

Avoiding the hay fever-causing allergen is obviously the best cure. If you know you get an allergy from particular plant pollen, try to keep it out of your house or your car. Because this is not always easy, pharmaceutical companies sell various over-the-counter and prescription medicines for the hay fever sufferer. Antihistamine is the most common. As the name suggests, antihistamine suppresses the release of cell histamine so that swelling and irritation is reduced. Medication that reduces the symptoms of the common cold, such as decongestants, also bring relief to hay fever symptoms.

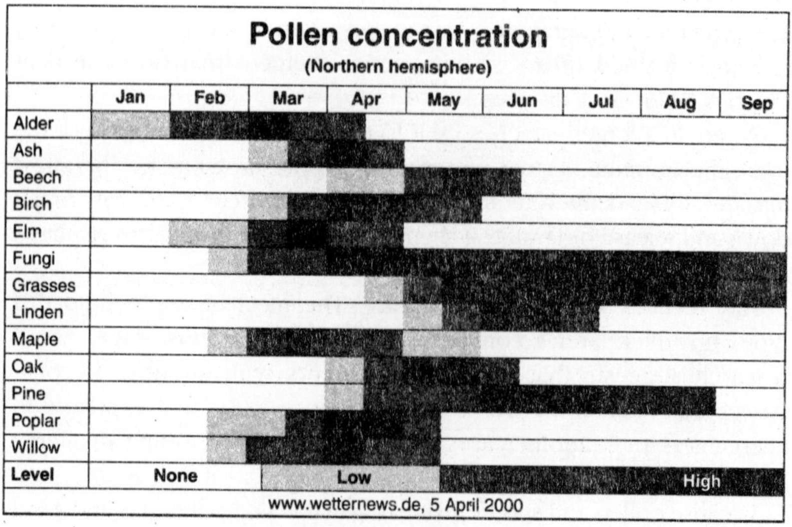

Asthma

Asthma is another burden for people in the so-called developed nations. The 'western' lifestyle is one of the possible causes that researchers presently investigate. Between 5% and 10% of US, Canadian, German, British and Australian citizens suffer from this debilitating and sometimes deadly disease—about half of them are children. The dramatic increase in numbers of asthma sufferers in recent years is of great concern. Throughout the world, the cases have doubled in the last 15 years, although a proportion of this increase is due to a growing awareness of the disease amongst patients and health professionals.

Asthma Triggers

- Allergens
- Exercise
- Weather
- Pollution
- Medical Conditions
- Food
- Medication

Your mother always told you not to speak with your mouth full and, if you just ignored the advice, a bit of food might have entered your airways. Automatically, your airways narrowed to prevent the substance from sliding further into the lung and you eventually coughed out the intruder. That is a normal reaction to a chunk of carrot. The lungs of asthmatics, however, overreact to mostly harmless triggers. The muscles around the airways spasmodically constrict and forget to relax. Breathing becomes very difficult during such an overreaction and may result in a medical emergency.

From here on, the body reactions are very similar to those of bronchitis and hay fever—the immune system combats the intruder. The airways become inflamed and mucus narrows or blocks bronchial tubes. Episodes of wheezing, coughing and shortness of breath plague the patient. Doctors often mistake acute bronchitis for asthma and vice versa. Asthma diagnosis becomes even more challenging when other diseases, such as hay fever and sinusitis, are present. The number of hay fever cases is several times greater amongst asthma patients.

Patients and their family members often underestimate the disease as well. Asthma often improves for a period of time and patients become complacent. A mild asthma attack, however, can progress to a life-threatening state within minutes. With proper emergency treatment, the disease is seldom deadly. But for more than 5,000 US citizens in 1995 and 685 Australians in 1999, the help arrived too late.

The mechanisms that cause asthma are still under intense investigation. So far, doctors can only treat the symptoms of asthma but can't cure it. Nevertheless, most substances or circumstances that trigger asthma are known.

Allergens are a common trigger of asthma. A patient reacts to one of many environmental substances, such as pollen, dust mites and pet hairs. The drying of the airways, as it occurs during vigorous exercise, is another common trigger, especially in children. Other factors are hereditary causes, medical conditions, pollution, food, medication and, of course, the weather.

Weather plays an important part in the life of an asthmatic. Winds collect and spread many types of allergens over large areas. The seasons determine the type of pollens and spores in the air. Cold weather keeps you inside where you are subjected to household and pet allergens. Inversions trap pollutants that cause asthma attacks. Low humidity makes the airways wheeze even more.

A morning with blue sky and fresh, crisp air heralds the beginning of a perfect autumn day—and is another example of a 'fine' day that is not fine for everybody. Hospital administrators can tell you that admissions of asthma patients may double during those days. Cold air causes the bronchial tubes to constrict, making breathing more difficult.

When a cold air mass comes from the inland, it is also very likely dry. The airways of children playing outside, or of people working and exercising outdoors, also dry out very quickly and become irritated. The combination of cooling and drying of the bronchial tubes is a major trigger of severe asthma attacks.

Pollution is a factor during spring and summer. Stagnant warm air contains a variety of chemical and organic pollutants. Sulphur dioxide, nitrogen dioxide, diesel fumes, particulate matter and ozone are all associated with asthma outbreaks. Ozone, in particular, adversely affects asthmatics, sometimes at levels below a nominated 'safe' standard.

I have already mentioned that rain and lightning significantly increase the presence of pollen allergens in the air. Researchers all over the world have found clear links between thunderstorm activities and asthma hospital admissions. In 1994, emergency department admissions in

12 London hospitals recorded a 10-fold increase in patient numbers with asthma and other respiratory problems after thunderstorms.

Asthma sufferers have two basic steps to treating their condition: remove the trigger and treat the symptoms. A multitude of medicines, mainly airways relaxants, is available to bring relief to patients. But finding the trigger is not always easy and removing it can be even more difficult, if not impossible. In addition, researchers found recently that certain circumstances, e.g. stress and obesity, aggravate asthma conditions. On the other hand, fitness and a healthy diet should help to ease the symptoms.

Infectious diseases

As if toxic pollution isn't enough, every breath you take fills your lungs with a multitude of dangerous germs. The sneeze of the person next to you, or the gases from animal housing nearby propels bacteria, viruses and fungi into the atmosphere. Natural or man-made turbulence lifts germs off the ground and into the breeze. Their survival depends largely on temperature, humidity and UV radiation.

Bacteria are the dominant life form on earth and adapt to almost all habitats. In the air they like to attach to other substances, thus increasing their chances of survival. Bacteria are present high in the atmosphere and drift long distances in the prevailing winds. Food and water are also likely carriers of bacteria. Most bacteria are harmless but others cause diseases such as cholera, pneumonia, leprosy, diphtheria, scarlet fever and tetanus.

Viruses don't feel as comfortable in the air as bacteria do. They require a host to multiply and most don't defend well against climatic variations and UV radiation. There are always exceptions, of course, such as the polio virus, which can live long enough to travel several kilometres. Some animal viral diseases can cause outbreaks from some distance away. Nevertheless, close contact is still the major means of spreading viral diseases such as chickenpox, influenza, measles and the common cold.

A major fungal disease dispersed by the air is histoplasmosis, also known as 'bird fever.' The fungus grows in bird and bat droppings. Dry droppings readily release the fungus into the air when they are disturbed, and then an unsuspecting person downwind inhales the microscopic organism and gets infected. While the lungs are the primary targets, the fungus can also invade other parts of the body. A mild attack has symptoms that are almost indistinguishable from those of the common cold, while a more serious form infects the liver and the eye.

The skin and the linings of nose, throat and airways are the first line of defence against any dangerous organism. When the immune system is impaired or the mucus layer is dry, the invaders break through the barrier and infect the tissue or enter the bloodstream. A bodily reaction to the invasion can occur at the point of entry or at a distant organ.

Chapter Four

Heat

Blame the heat for:

- Food poisoning
- Heat rash
- Heat cramps
- Muscle meltdown
- Heatstroke
- Dehydration

and more

Introduction

The sun's heat radiation is the basis for life on this planet. Without it, none would exist. Radiant heat from the sun, either direct or reflected, warms your body. To a degree, your body generates some of its own heat—through its metabolism. Last night's steak is still 'warming' your body and just reading this paragraph creates heat in your brain. The muscles create heat, even while sitting still, but exercise or hard work generates up to twenty times more. As with everything else though, you can have too much of a good thing.

When the temperature rises too much, discomfort and illness develop. Heat-related illnesses range from minor disorders, like swollen legs or heat rash, to the more serious and dangerous conditions of dehydration and heatstroke. The elderly, the very young and the sick are at greatest risk. Although it could be prevented, many thousands of people die each year as a direct or indirect result of heat-related illnesses.

What is Heat?

'The children are full of energy today.' That's what you say whenever they are madly running around. Similarly, the molecules and atoms of a hot substance hop and dance or vibrate tirelessly. This activity is energy and heat is a form of energy. Not only do hot substances contain heat, even the tiny particles in an ice cube similarly jig up and down, although their activity level is very low. The cube does not contain much energy (heat)—it is said to be cold.

Heat energy doesn't like to be confined. Like water, heat flows from a source with an abundance of it to somewhere with less—heat is thus transferred. This can happen in four ways: radiation, conduction, convection and evaporation.

Radiation is the process of heat transfer without going through a carrier substance. The sun transmits heat in such a way, through the emptiness of outer space. Stand in the sun and you can feel the radiation on your skin. Of course, this works the other way as well. Your body constantly radiates heat to the surroundings and thereby loses heat.

Conduction is heat transfer by contact. Touch a hot oven and an immense amount of heat energy transfers into your palm. If you don't want to admit your foolishness just say, 'I was part of the conduction process between an oven's hot plate and the palm of my hand', which sounds so much better than, 'I damned well burnt my hand!' But by the same principle, an ice cube in your hand feels cold because your body transfers heat energy to the cube.

When the sun heats the roofs of city buildings, the air above them also becomes hot. It is then lighter than the surrounding cooler air, so it rises. This rising air carries heat energy into the atmosphere. The process of moving heat within a gas or liquid is called convection.

Heat energy is required to evaporate water. To boil water for a cup of coffee requires a significant amount of energy. Even more energy is needed to turn some of the water into water vapour. This extra energy to create the vapour isn't lost, however, it's stored in the vapour; it is latent. When the vapour condenses, i.e. the steam turns into water droplets, the energy originally needed to form the gas is released again in the form of heat. Clouds, in particular thunderstorm clouds, contain an immense amount of heat energy. In other words, the expensive energy you bought from the power or gas company is wasted to evaporate some of the water in your coffee kettle, and the vapour will travel across your backyard fence until it reaches a suitable place where it can condense again. There it releases the same amount of energy that you put in. Not fair, is it?

What is Temperature?

Temperature measures the flow of heat energy from one substance to another. For example, if you hold a thermometer in warm water, heat energy flows from the water to the cool thermometer. If we use a mercury-filled thermometer, the increasingly active mercury atoms need more room to move, and make the liquid mercury expand. Once the mercury atoms reaches the same level of activity as those of the warm water, the expansion stops. And we notice the mercury settle next to a temperature reading that corresponds with that of the water.

Fahrenheit versus Celsius

Temperature	Fahrenheit	Celsius
Absolute zero	–459.67	–273.15
Zero Fahrenheit	0.0	–17.8
Freezing point of water	32.0	0.0
Body temperature	98.4	36.9
100 degrees Fahrenheit	100.0	37.8
Boiling point of water	212.0	100.0

Temperature Conversion

°C = χ°F – 32 x 5/9

°F = χ°C + 32 x 9/5

Different types of temperature scales are in use. Worldwide the most popular is the Celsius scale, where 0°C is the freezing point of water and 100°C the boiling point. The Fahrenheit scale, still used in the US, shows 32°F as the freezing point and 212°F as the boiling point. Another scale worth mentioning is the Kelvin scale, also known as the Absolute scale. Zero degree Kelvin is equal to the lowest possible temperature, which is –273.15°C. At this temperature, no molecular or atomic activity takes place, so there is no heat.

To get a fair comparison between the temperatures of two different locations, meteorologists standardize where and when they take their measurements. It isn't reliable to take one measurement at high noon, in full sun and near a brick wall and compare it with another taken in the morning shade under a tree. To be able to compare temperatures worldwide, meteorological offices all measure temperatures at the same time of the day and in the shade of a purpose-built instrument shelter.

Highest recorded temperatures

Continent	Temp. (deg C)	Temp. (deg F)	Place	Date
Africa	58	136.5	El Azizia, Libya	13 Sep 1922
N. America	57	134.5	Death Valley, US, California	10 Jul 1913
Asia	54	129	Tirat Tsvi, Israel	21 Jun 1942
Australia	53	127.5	Cloncurry, Queensland	16 Jan 1889
Europe	50	122	Seville, Spain	4 Aug 1881
S. America	49	120	Rivadavia, Argentina	11 Dec 1905

HEAT AND THE BODY

Body temperature

Humans survive in the extreme cold of the polar region and the hot and humid conditions of the equatorial tropics. Despite the climatic variety of the habitats we occupy, our core body remains at approximately 36.9°C. Even someone acclimatized to the polar regions has an average core body temperature only 0.2°C lower than a person living in the tropics.

Our insides and our brain don't like to depart much from the average, either. We can feel stressed as soon as the temperature rises or falls by more than one degree, and feel the need to add or remove clothing, seek shelter, or switch on a heater or cooler. Meanwhile, the body's own temperature control mechanism goes into action.

Hypothalamus

A tiny gland that weighs less than 4g drives your sex life. It may seem disappointing, but it's true. The hypothalamus, located in the centre of the brain at the top of the brain stem, also controls your behaviour, the metabolic process, emotions, the involuntary (autonomic) nervous system and the systems that regulate your body temperature.

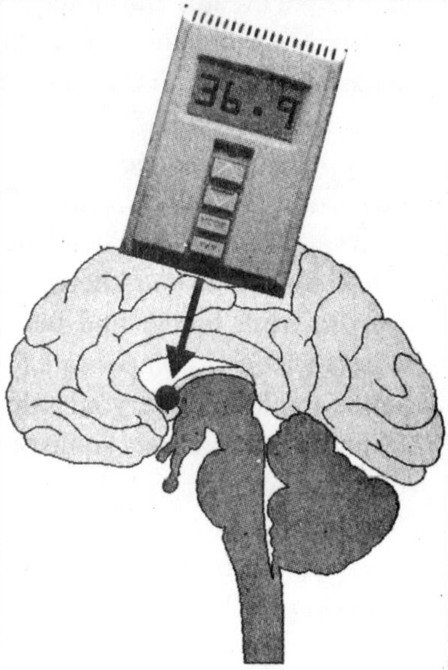

Hypothalamus
The Body's Thermostat

The hypothalamus responds to any rise or drop in body temperature by releasing a particular hormone. This contains instructions for the body to sweat or shiver, contract or expand blood vessels, and increase or decrease the heartbeat and breathing rate. The hypothalamus detects thermal comfort or discomfort and tells you that it is time to escape from the heat or button up against the cold.

As with all of our other body parts, this gland is not perfect—an accident, stroke, disease or tumour can impair its function. When we are born, the hypothalamus isn't fully developed and its functions degenerate with age, so that the very young, the elderly and people with a disease affecting the hypothalamus are particularly vulnerable to temperature extremes.

Heat loss

Your internal organs digest the food you eat. This process creates heat. Without systems to shed some of this heat, the body temperature would rise too high. The systems are:

- **Breathing.** You need to breathe in oxygen to aid the process of burning calories. At the same time, the hot air in the lungs is replaced with cooler air from outside, thus cooling your body. What happens on a hot day when the outside air is warmer than the air in the lungs? There is another process happening at the same time—evaporation.

  The moisture in your lungs converts to water vapour through evaporation, but this can only take place if the air is not already saturated with vapour. Breathing, therefore, will do very little to cool down your body if you breathe hot and humid air. Under normal circumstances we breathe through the nose and if this isn't enough to cool the body, we breathe or pant through the mouth.
- **Circulation.** The blood carries a large amount of heat to all parts of the body, including the skin. On the surface of the skin three other forms of heat exchange other than evaporation take place—radiation, convection and conduction.

  During hot days or while exercising, the normal blood circulation is not sufficient. Our thermostat, the hypothalamus, instructs the heart to work harder and beat faster. At the same time, the blood vessels widen to compensate for the increased blood flow. You will notice a reddening of your skin.

  The hot skin radiates some of the excess energy into the surroundings. The hot air near your skin rises, thus carrying energy away from your body, a process called convection. Dip into the pool, and you lose even more through conduction.
- **Sweating.** When exposed to temperatures below 20°C, the body loses most of its heat through radiation and conduction. Above this temperature, evaporation through sweating begins to aid the heat transfer. Two to five million sweat glands in your skin will open on command and shed great quantities of water. A person exercising and sweating profusely dissipates three-quarters of their body heat and can lose up to two litres of water per hour. Top athletes become miniature waterfalls that can shed up to three litres per hour.

  The rate of heat loss through sweating is very much determined by the surrounding air's humidity. If the air is already saturated, or contains a large amount of water vapour, sweat won't or will only slowly evaporate. Non-porous clothing will further hinder evaporation. Sweat contains essential body salts (electrolytes), and excess perspiration can severely disrupt their balance in the body, and lead to certain medical conditions.

See Chapter Five, 'Cold', for more information on conduction, convection, radiation and evaporation.

Heat disorders develop when the three cooling systems are insufficient to keep your body temperature at its normal level. A body temperature rise above 41°C causes weakness or exhaustion. A further rise to levels above 42.5°C may result in serious health problems or even death.

Acclimatization

You step from the aircraft on to the tarmac where the heat and humidity hits you like a sledgehammer. If you had a knife you could carve the air. The legs are heavy like lead, almost as heavy as the sweat-soaked clothes. Why did you think of fleeing the bitter winter and accepting a job in this tropical country? It's really no problem eventually; you acclimatize.

The process stresses your body, though. For the first few days you probably feel exhausted and your work performance suffers. A healthy person requires up to 14 days to fully acclimatize. In the first week, your cardiovascular system adapts slowly: your blood volume increases by up to 20% and your heart rate decreases by between 15% to 25%. This is a temporary adjustment and should normalize by the end of two weeks.

Long-term adaptations include an improved ability to lose heat more efficiently. The blood flow to the skin increases, aiding heat loss due to radiation, convection and conduction. Dormant sweat glands become active and increase the sweat rate. The

Physiological responses to heat

- Activation of dormant sweat glands
- Increased blood flow to skin
- More efficient heat dissipation
- Increased blood volume
- Decrease in heart rate
- Altered metabolism.

sweat, however, is less salty because the kidneys learn to prevent excessive loss of electrolytes. Your metabolism also changes. It limits the process of calorie burning, thus reducing heat generation.

Luckily, you can use your brain to assist the body—and choose to consume cooling food and drink during long exposure to heat. A low-calorie diet means fewer calories to burn. Of course, wearing appropriate clothing is another major factor—you won't need the fur coat in Hawaii.

Unfortunately, you lose the benefits of acclimatization very quickly when you return to the previous climatic conditions. All the hard work vanishes within a few days.

Risk factors

Excessive heat affects everybody. Certain age groups, conditions and activities, however, will pose a higher risk of developing heat-related illnesses. The following list provides some examples, but is not exhaustive:

- **Children.** In infants, the hypothalamus, and its heat regulation mechanism, is underdeveloped, while their sweat glands are small and operate less efficiently. Less blood flows to the outer skin and children acclimatize slower. Their metabolism creates more heat as compared to an adult performing the same amount of activity.
- **The aged.** The hypothalamus degenerates with age, so that the heat regulation mechanism responds slower to body signals. Sweating and blood circulation becomes less efficient. The elderly end up with a diminished sense of thirst and, as a consequence, may not take in enough fluid. In addition, the elderly have more chronic conditions and are more often forced to remain in bed or at home during hot conditions.
- **Obesity.** Fatty tissue blocks sweat glands and impairs blood circulation in the skin. Also, a layer of body fat acts as an insulator and traps heat.
- **Excessive physical activity.** An athlete or outdoor worker can lose up to three litres of sweat per hour. Unfortunately, the person can't replace this amount immediately, as the body only absorbs approximately one litre of imbibed liquid per hour. The net loss leads to dehydration.

- **Medical conditions.** Underlying health problems will increase the risk of heat-related illnesses. For example:
  - High blood pressure (hypertension)
  - Diabetes
  - Damaged or diseased skin
  - Diseased heart or blood vessels (cardiovascular disease)
  - Fever
  - Excess of thyroid hormones, increased metabolic rate (hyperthyroidism).
- **Medication and drugs** can increase the body's stress level during heat, which is undesirable if there's a risk of dehydration. Antihistamines and some tranquillizers can interfere with sweating. Beverages such as tea, coffee and alcohol are diuretic, meaning they stimulate the body to loose fluid. Recent findings show that the combination of heat and the use of recreational drugs can also lead to fatalities.
- **Other factors.** The lack of air conditioning and unsuitable housing or work environments will exacerbate heat wave effects. Some workers or athletes have to wear heavy protective clothing despite unfavourable environmental conditions.

Medications contributing to the risk of heat illnesses

Alpha agonists	Heroin
Amphetamines	Inhaled anaesthetics
Anticholinergic medications	Laxatives
Antihistamines	LSD
Anti-Parkinsonian agents	Monoamine oxidase inhibitors
Beta-blockers	Phencyclidine
Calcium channel blockers	Phenothiazines
Cocaine	Sympathomimetic medications
Diuretics	Thyroid agonists
Ethanol	Tricyclic antidepressants

American Academy of Family Physicians (1 September 1998)

Heat index

We can tolerate hot and dry conditions better than hot and humid conditions. On humid days the air 'feels' hotter than it actually is, and vice versa on dry days. This apparent temperature is based on relative humidity and air temperature.

For easy use, the US National Weather Service developed an internationally recognized heat index table. The creators of the index assume that you are in the shade and there is no wind. For example, an air temperature of 30°C has the effect of 41°C when the relative humidity is at around 90%. Temperatures in direct sunlight are up to 8°C higher.

Heat index table – Celsius

	Air temperature								
	28	**29**	**30**	**31**	**32**	**33**	**34**	**35**	**36**
Humidity	**Apparent temperature**								
50%	28	30	31	33	34	36	38	40	43
60%	29	31	33	35	37	39	42	45	48
70%	31	33	35	38	40	43	47	50	54
80%	32	35	38	41	44	48	52	56	61
90%	34	37	41	45	49	53	58	64	69

HEAT-RELATED DISORDERS

Skill impairment

You parked your car in the sun for just a short while. Nevertheless, the interior temperature quickly climbed to 65°C or above, enough to melt that favourite music cassette you left on the dashboard. You drive off and the car's air conditioner slowly becomes effective. The large glass windows, however, can't prevent the sun's radiation heating parts of your body. You feel very uncomfortable. On top of that, a spate of road accidents reduced the traffic to a crawl—the other drivers are all idiots. Didn't you just miss a red light?

An early sign of heat stress is tiredness, exhaustion or irritability. Any physical or mental task becomes stressful and the performance suffers. Tests of workers with different skills established that the accuracy in physical and mental tasks drops quite markedly even at relatively mild temperatures between 28.5°C and 31°C. Temperatures of 32°C and above led to a notable decrease in short-term memory. In an audio vigilance test, Morse code operators made significantly more errors with increasing temperatures. Underground mine workers have to endure high temperatures and humidity. Performance suffers as follows:

- A loss of body weight of around 2% due to sweating results in a work rate dropping by up to 7%
- A weight loss of 4% dramatically lowers the work rate by between 22% and 50%
- Mental performance decreases as dehydration increases above 2%.

Results of examinations performed by students in air conditioned classrooms are significantly better than the results of students who completed the same exams in a warm environment. But despite air conditioning, body temperatures of military pilots rose by up to 2°C during flight and while exposed to the sun's radiation under Perspex-canopied cockpits. That is like flying with a fever. Simple tasks are no longer simple. Pilots miss checklist items, flick the wrong switches and violate rules and regulations. Even with a comfortable cockpit temperature, an elevated body temperature just prior a flight can take up to 30 minutes to reach normal levels.

To blame violent crime on the weather appears to be far-fetched. Statistical evidence, however, associates a rise in numbers of assault, robbery, domestic violence and rape with temperature increases. Hot-blooded?

Conception and birth

Enough evidence is mounting to substantiate a direct link between heat and sperm quality and quantity. Exposure to excessive heat invariably leads to an elevated testicular temperature. As a result, sperm often becomes deformed (tapered), lacks the ability to propel itself, and/or is missing the acrosome, a granule at the tip of the sperm that releases a substance on contact with an egg to facilitate entry into it. Sperm quality deteriorates substantially during the summer months.

Women can't entirely blame men for low conception rates during hot weather conditions. Fertility-related female hormones may also be affected by temperature extremes.

Where fertility and conception is an issue, men should prevent exposure to heat and wear loose underpants. Now there's an idea for a new enterprise. But 'air-conditioned' underwear is already available. Scientists at Melbourne's Monash University in Australia teamed up with the industry to develop and produce cool and sperm-friendly boxer shorts. 'The key factor is heat. Boxer shorts, which permit air flow in the testicular region, keep the testes cooler—which aids healthy sperm production and helps to prevent reproductive problems such as male infertility,' Professor David de Kretser said. The final product is a cotton boxer short with a mesh brief that provides coolness and support.

Food poisoning

Another scorcher of a day is forecast and bacteria such as salmonella, *E. coli* and staphylococci just love it. These tiny organisms thrive and multiply in warm conditions. Most grow at temperatures between 5 and 60°C but are particularly active at the halfway mark. In this temperature range, the bacteria chew away on their piece of chicken, meat, fish, or any other food and leave their toxic excrement for you to eat. You may develop stomach cramps, diarrhoea or vomiting. Temperatures above 60°C kill bacteria, but their residues remain toxic.

The victims often don't report mild cases of food poisoning, and if they do the doctor may attribute the symptoms to some other disease. The true number of food poisoning victims, therefore, can only be estimated. US government officials believe that between 24 and 81 million cases of diarrhoea occur every year as a result of food-borne bacteria, at a cost of between $A10 and $A34 billion to the community (medical care and lost productivity). In the UK, some 2 million people suffer from food poisoning every year, where hot spells result in a massive increase in food poisoning incidents: every degree the temperature goes up, the incidents rise by 7%.

The future doesn't look good either. The Centre for Social and Economic Research in the UK predicts an additional 179,000 cases of food poisoning by the year 2050 if global warming takes its expected effect.

While death as a direct result of food poisoning is rare, the combination of its symptoms with other factors such as heat-related illnesses, immune system deficiency and other diseases can be enough to cause the mortality rate to increase during an outbreak. One estimate puts the figure at 9,000 US citizens per year.

The cook is often the first person to take the wrath of a diarrhoea-riddled consumer. But the contamination can take place at any stage in the farming, distribution and preparation process. Almost all contamination is a result of improper food handling in commercial and industrial establishments. Only about a fifth of contamination occurs at home. The increasing reliance on take-away food, catering services, restaurants, institutional kitchens and convenience food increases the risk of mass outbreaks of food-borne illnesses.

The weather is only indirectly to blame for an outbreak. Food providers will have to take in consideration a forecasted hot spell and adjust their food handling practices accordingly.

Blood pressure

Your blood vessels widen with rising temperature to let more blood flow to the skin. The heart needs then to apply less pressure to pump the same amount of blood through the vessels—so the blood pressure falls. A comparison between outside air temperatures and the blood pressure of blood donors reveals an average 10–15% lower blood pressure during the warmer months of the year and an increase by the same amount during the colder winter months.

This sounds good for people with high blood pressure. Keep in mind, however, that when the body needs to shed excess heat, the pulse rate increases dramatically and puts the heart under considerable strain. Physical exertion in combination with an underlying heart disease is a major contributor to high death rates during heat waves.

Swollen legs

After many hours sitting on an overseas flight you may find that your shoes have shrunk. They didn't, of course—your legs have swollen.

When you walk, the muscles in your legs repeatedly pressure the blood vessels, thereby pumping some of the blood up towards the heart. Without the muscle movements, as during prolonged sitting or standing, fluid will exit the blood vessels and pool in your legs, making them swell.

Although not quite as severely, the same problem can arise in your hands. Heat worsens the situation. Blood vessels widen when exposed to high temperatures and more fluid remains in your extremities.

Immobility and heat are two major causes for the swelling, or fluid retention (oedema). Others include the use of certain medication, diet, hormone changes during pregnancy, and a hereditary condition called lipedema. The swelling can also indicate a more serious problem, because blocked blood vessels and lymph channels, infections and tumours affect the blood flow and cause fluid retention. Exercising the muscles and cooling the affected area are the easiest ways to treat the condition.

Heat intolerance

'I hate the heat.' No, this is not heat intolerance. Heat intolerance is an illness that impairs the normal functions of the body's temperature regulation system. Even the slightest rise in temperature triggers hot flushes and profuse sweating in some patients. Normally, your body adapts to hot conditions (see 'Acclimatization' p. 57), but someone with heat intolerance doesn't adapt, or does so very slowly.

One common cause is the excess hormone production of the thyroid gland—a condition known as hyperthyroidism. Too much of the hormone increases the metabolic rate, which creates more heat. Exercise and medication can aggravate hyperthyroidism, so if you have the condition you should maintain a comfortable room temperature and replenish lost fluid.

Heat rash

The purpose of sweat is to evaporate and cool your body. Wearing non-porous covers, such as plastic baby diapers, oily make-up or tight-fitting garments, however, will hold the sweat within the glands. This may lead to an irritation of the glands and the formation of small red pimples or even blisters—symptoms of heat rash. It isn't generally serious, but can develop into a secondary skin infection. Hot and humid weather is almost always the cause, but obesity, genetic factors and sensitive skin also add to your chances of heat rash.

Heat rash—also known as prickly heat and baby rash—is more common amongst the very young, because their underdeveloped sweat glands clog easily. Even in winter an overdressed infant in a wet diaper can develop the pimples between the legs and on the buttocks.

Prevent heat rash by removing the cause of the sweat gland blockage. Don't wear tight-fitting and non-porous garments in the summer heat. Avoid oily ointments and creams where possible and wash off any sweat or dirt. Change baby diapers regularly and apply moisture-absorbing powder. If prevention comes too late, your pharmacy has antiseptic cleansers or soothing remedies.

Although heat rash is a non-serious and common medical condition in babies, it is also a sign that the infant is too hot, and may progress to a more dangerous heat-related disorder.

Heat cramps

Sweating excessively without replacing the lost fluid results in dehydration and an imbalance of body salt levels (electrolytes). As a consequence, painful cramps in the major muscles develop rapidly, but sometimes not until several hours after the event. Especially vulnerable are the hamstrings of your legs and the muscles of your arms and stomach. They become hard and painfully tense and often disable the affected person.

Electrolytes are chemicals that make fluids electrically conductive. You probably heard the term in relation to your car battery. The mechanic replenishes the electrolyte, in this case battery acid, when it is too low. Without electrolyte you wouldn't have an electric current—your engine wouldn't start. The body, too, requires electrolytes. Besides their conductive properties, body salts regulate the fluid levels in the body cells and control the function of the kidneys. The two major chemicals acting as electrolytes in the body fluids are sodium (table salt) and potassium.

After heavy sweating, replenish yourself with water and electrolytes. Half a teaspoon of salt dissolved in each litre of water is generally sufficient to top up the electrolyte levels. Sports drinks, or salty food together with water, are similarly effective. Rest in a cool place, out of the sun, to avoid a deterioration of the condition. See a doctor if you also have symptoms (see below) of heat exhaustion or heatstroke.

Heat exhaustion

The cause of heat exhaustion is similar to that of heat cramp—dehydration and/or an imbalance of body salts. In this case, however, the body's temperature regulation system fails to adequately respond to an increase in body temperature as well. The disorder often follows overexertion in hot weather during sport or outdoor work. Elderly patients on diuretic medicines are also at great risk.

The signs and symptoms are similar to shock and include:

- Weakness, exhaustion, fatigue
- Nausea and vomiting
- Diarrhoea
- Heat cramps
- Lack of coordination, giddiness, faintness
- Rapid pulse and breathing
- Cold and clammy skin
- Profuse sweating.

Someone showing these symptoms should be moved to a cool place, have their unnecessary garments removed and their body cooled. Lost fluids and electrolytes should be replaced. Consult a doctor if the person can't keep the fluid down or doesn't recover promptly. The condition is very similar to heatstroke, but the body temperature is usually less than 39°C.

Heat syncope

This condition is a temporary loss of consciousness, or fainting, triggered by prolonged standing in the heat. The dilated blood vessels allow the blood to pool in the otherwise stationary lower parts of the body.

If someone is unable or unwilling to move their legs, the brain suffers temporarily a shortage of blood—and fainting occurs. A horizontal body position aids the blood flow to the brain and the situation corrects itself within minutes.

Heat syncope occurrences during parades of soldiers or the police are a typical example. As fit as most of them are, standing still in hot conditions and enduring boring speeches or presentations fells even the toughest. And a felling it is. Without much warning, the person faints and hits the ground. He or she will wake up in the arms of a caring ambulance officer. Unfortunately, not only the ego may be bruised.

Muscle meltdown

Another marathon runner breaks down at the finishing line and is rushed to the hospital for treatment. Chances are that the athlete has overheated some muscles and suffers from a potentially life-threatening muscle meltdown. 'I'm not a marathon runner, so why should I care?' you say. Unfortunately, the illness is quite common. Rhabdomyolisis, as it is known to doctors, may strike by itself or can coexist with other heat-related illnesses, such as heat intolerance or heatstroke. Estimates put its occurrence at 1 in 10,000 people, regardless of age or gender. Untrained or non-acclimatized people exerting themselves in hot and humid weather are potential victims.

When the muscles overheat, they accumulate large amounts of calcium in their cells. This activates enzymes, which in turn kills the cells. The residue of the cells is then released into the bloodstream and filtered out by the kidneys. One compound of the dead cells is myoglobin. Just as cholesterol can congest your blood vessels, myoglobin clogs up the fine canals in the kidneys. Once the myoglobin breaks down, it becomes toxic. Both effects, the clogging and the toxicity, may lead to kidney damage or failure.

Dehydration

You survive for days and weeks without food, but you will last only hours without water in extreme heat. You don't have to be stranded in a desert to become dehydrated, either. Just digging the vegetable patch, or working and exercising on a hot day can result in excess fluid loss.

Dehydration is defined as the loss of water and/or electrolytes from the body without adequate replenishment. Everyone loses more than one litre of fluid per day in urine and faeces, their breath, and in mild sweat, despite not lifting a finger. You can lose up to two litres of fluid per hour if you work hard and sweat profusely. You drain your body even further if you vomit or get an attack of diarrhoea. If you lose between 5% and 10% of your body fluid, you have mild to moderate dehydration. Once the loss reaches 15% or more, however, severe damage to body organs is likely.

'I'm thirsty.' Dehydration's first warning sign is a craving—thirst—for anything liquid. This mechanism, however, is unreliable. But if the body loses a very high proportion of salts, the craving for liquids diminishes or is not apparent at all. In old age you have also an inhibited appreciation of thirst.

Other warning signs are headaches, dry lips and mouth, loss of concentration, fatigue, and dry and wrinkled skin. The appearance of large amounts of sweat is normally another caution that you should drink something. But this visual check is sometimes misleading. On very dry and hot days, the sweat evaporates so fast that it doesn't form sweat pearls on the skin. Once dehydration progresses, the body gradually loses weight.

The body releases a specific hormone (vasopressin) when the fluid level becomes too low. The hormone is a chemical signal for the kidneys to preserve water by reducing urine production. This can go too far. The body's waste, normally extracted by the kidneys, accumulates in the blood and causes poisoning. If the fluid level continues to drop despite the effort to preserve water, the kidneys lose their function altogether—kidney failure occurs.

Low fluid levels lead to the failure of the cooling mechanisms; you can't sweat if you don't have enough fluid in your body. In addition, if the blood volume decreases, it carries less heat to the skin for dissipation. As a consequence, dehydration causes overheating.

So, you better fill up your reservoirs. But remember coffee, tea and alcohol increase the urine production and dehydrate you even further. Some diuretic medications accelerate the loss of body fluids as well. For the elderly, the combination of heavy sweating, diuretics and an impaired thirst sensation is dangerous.

Always drink more than you 'think' you should. If you trust your thirst, you won't fill up enough, as thirst generally stops when you've replenished about two-thirds of the lost fluids. While sweating you lose a large amount of electrolytes, so see 'Heat Cramps' for tips on how to top up electrolyte levels.

Professional athletes competing in hot conditions take preventive measures. They drink fluids in advance—they prehydrate. In addition, they ensure they drink the right amount after the competition to compensate for the loss of body weight.

Heatstroke

Heatstroke is the most dangerous of all heat-related illnesses and requires immediate medical attention. I have previously explained the limitations of the body's ability to regulate its temperature. When the self-cooling process is stressed beyond its capabilities, it may collapse completely. The condition becomes life threatening and, despite medical attention, approximately 10% of heatstroke patients die. The rate is much higher during heat wave conditions or in regions where medical help is limited.

A healthy person is not likely to succumb to heat and high humidity unless that person increases their body temperature during work or exercise in hot conditions. The elderly and the very young with a deficient or underdeveloped heat regulation mechanism, however, are always at risk to suffer from heatstroke, with or without physical activity. Chronic illnesses, genetic makeup and some types of medication can also increase the risk.

The signs and symptoms of heatstroke are:

- Body temperature climbs to 40.5°C or higher
- Headache
- Nausea, vomiting
- Visual disturbances
- Altered mental state whereby dizziness, irritability, confusion, progression to seizures and unconsciousness is possible
- Rapid pulse
- Flushed and usually dry skin. Sweat can be present in exertional heatstroke.

Recognition of heatstroke symptoms is vital to allow prompt medical attention. If the patient isn't cooled immediately, the high body temperature will damage the tissue of almost every organ. Muscle meltdown (rhabdomyolisis) and blood clotting (thrombosis) often accompany heatstroke.

A survey of several heatstroke patients showed that all suffered from multiorgan dysfunction. About half had kidney problems and showed symptoms of blood clotting. More than half had breathing difficulties and required intubation, where a tube was inserted to help them breathe. Most survivors recovered to almost normal conditions, but a third were left with permanent organ or brain damage.

Sunstroke

Your bald-headed guest turns more and more red. But you are sure he isn't ashamed of the dirty joke you just told him. Now he even runs to the toilet with an urge to vomit. But you told him this joke many times and he never reacted with such disgust! Was it the burnt sausage he took from the barbecue? Blame the weather. Your guest has classical symptoms of sunstroke.

The term sunstroke is often used in place of heatstroke. Heatstroke is an overexposure to heat, no matter whether you are in the sun, the shade, or indoors. Sunstroke, on the other hand, is caused by overexposure to the sun's radiation. Direct radiation to an unprotected head with sparse or no hair cover penetrates the skull and irritates the outer layers of the brain. At the same time, the head overheats if the blood circulation is insufficient to carry the excess heat away. Babies are at particular risk. Their skull is still very thin and membranes are the only cover for the openings between the bony structures (fontanelle).

The victim often has a hot and flushed head accompanied by headache, nausea, dizziness and irritability. If the person does the sensible thing and moves into the shade, the symptoms disappear quickly. If not, wet towels or air circulation should return the head to its normal temperature. Further exposure, however, can lead to expansion of the brain and damage to its cells. Severe headache, vomiting and unconsciousness may result. The situation becomes a medical emergency.

HEAT WAVE

How do we define a heat wave? The *Encyclopaedia Britannica* defines it simply as 'a period of exceptionally hot weather, often with high humidity'. But what is 'exceptionally hot'? For the occupants of Casey in the Antarctic, the highest recorded temperature of 9.2°C must have felt like an exceptionally hot day. By contrast, the population of Marble Bar, a small town in Australia's Pilbara region, may feel quite comfortable with their average daily maximum of above 40°C in summer. The town holds the infamous record of more than 170 consecutive days above 37.8°C. Despite these high temperatures, even the settlers of European descent think of it as nothing unusual—they are acclimatized.

Heat waves do have a much more dramatic effect on people living in a cool to mild climate. They experience a higher degree of stress to their bodies than acclimatized residents of subtropical and tropical regions do. For example, death rates in Great Britain and the Netherlands increase sharply when the thermometer climbs above 25°C.

Devastating heat waves in the last five years of the 20th century pose the question whether global warming has increased the frequency and

Heat wave headlines

Spain	July 1995	'13 deaths, Toledo hits 42.2°C'
US	Summer 1995	'Heat wave kills 1021 Americans'
Pakistan	June 1996	'Heat wave claims dozens of lives'
India	June 1998	'Already more than 2500 deaths in heat wave'
Europe	July 1998	'Devastating heat wave in the Mediterranean'
Cyprus	August 1998	'52 deaths during heat wave'
Israel	October 1998	'5000 Haifa residents evacuated'
Russia	July 1999	'Russians suffer from longest heat wave ever'
Sweden	August 1999	'Wildfire in Sweden'
US	August 1999	'Heat-related death toll hits 220'
Japan	August 1999	'At least 16 heat-related deaths in Japan'

severity of heat waves. There is no doubt that the earth is getting warmer. Highest ever temperatures are being recorded throughout the world. But many scientists are still not prepared to link these recent temperature extremes to global warming, as they say heat waves have been a fact of summer since recording started.

In the meantime, weather forecasting takes into account the impact of heat on human health. Weather services issue warnings whenever the temperature and humidity is expected to reach a certain level. Scientists developed an apparent temperature table: Heat Index. Community services issue emergency and educational messages through the media that deal with the health implications and prevention of heat-related illnesses. Employers agree to reduce the employee's workload or stop work altogether on hot days.

Mortality rate

Heat injures and kills, as we can see from the thousands of people who die of heat-related illnesses each year. In 1996, Pakistan and India experienced temperatures of up to 49°C in the shade; people died or were hospitalized for heatstroke, circulatory collapse or dehydration. The Indian press reported a death toll of 2,500, but acknowledged that the number was probably much higher. The US experienced two particularly disastrous years: according to the Centres of Disease Control and Prevention, 1,700 Americans died in 1980. The US National Weather Service reported 1,021 deaths in 1995. In the UK and the Netherlands, temperatures above 25°C appear to have a close relationship with death rates for most diseases, excepting cancer.

Depending on the research methods, the figures that each government agency publishes often conflict. They have to rely heavily on death certificates and/or hospital reports issued by a medical officer. But how do these medical professionals classify a heat-related death?

A person died of a heart attack. Did the heart surrender to the demand of the body's temperature control mechanism to pump large amounts of blood to the skin? Another person drank a considerable amount of alcohol during a hot day. Did the person die as a result of the toxic effect of alcohol, or due to a heatstroke? The heat most likely played a role in both cases. But would the person have lived under different circumstances? What was the primary cause?

These questions can lead to the speculation that the actual heat-related death toll is considerably under-reported. Critics suggest that the official figures should be up to twice as high but even as they currently stand, heat mortality rates are too high.

The media always seems to be preoccupied with death rates. We shouldn't forget the many victims left with permanent health damage. A lack of records makes it hard to determine the number of people who become ill. But for every dead person there must be many more survivors burdened with brain, kidney or liver damage. Some will become heat intolerant and will be in particular danger when the next heat wave comes around.

Economic and social impact

A long hot spell affects humans indirectly as well—at times, quite dramatically. Drought often accompanies a heat wave and agriculture is usually the first industry that suffers. Plants wilt in the sun. Livestock suffers heat stress. Irrigation water becomes scarce. As a consequence, productivity drops markedly.

On hot days with very low humidities, water evaporates at a rapid rate and limits the availability of drinking water. Heat waves lead to a considerable increase in demand for water and restrictions may be imposed. The shortage of clean drinking water during India's devastating heat wave in 1998 is partially to blame for the high death toll.

Despite the cooling effect of evaporation, the water temperature in lakes and rivers rises. The population of fish and waterborne insects are very sensitive to temperature changes, and they only survive within a very narrow temperature band and anything beyond means belly up—literally. But there is something that loves the warm water: algae. High water temperatures result in algae blooms. Despite being classified as a plant, there is nothing pretty about its bloom. It multiplies very quickly and chokes a lake or river to death.

Heat can severely interrupt transportation. Mechanical failures in trucks, cars, trains and buses are common in heat waves. Heavy traffic damages the softened asphalt on roads, leaving the community with expensive repairs. Even concrete buckles in extreme heat. Steel railroad tracks expand and distort once the expansion gaps are bridged. Hot air is thin and thin air creates less lift on aircraft wings, so the aircraft have to reduce their passenger or cargo load.

Air conditioning equipment requires a substantial amount of electricity to operate. Unfortunately, when the demand for electricity is greatest, the generators in power stations are often overburdened and the supply breaks down. Power lines expand and sag in extreme heat and may cause short circuits.

Fire requires fuel, oxygen and heat. During hot conditions, a tinder-dry forest is the fuel; the air contains the oxygen; the sun provides the heat. Every year bushfires kill hundreds of people and burn vast areas of forests, agricultural land and man-made structures. Smoke and toxic gases threaten the health of humans and animals.

Heat island effect

You sit on your shaded veranda and enjoy a cool drink. The sea breeze blows gently through the large open windows and coconut trees provide shade from the sun. Dream on: you are more likely one of the million city dwellers living in a brick or concrete bunker, built to save energy during frosty winter months. An environmentalist at heart, you installed small and double-glazed windows and insulated walls and ceiling. Good on you. To beat the summer heat, you rely on air conditioning—if you can afford it and if you have the electricity to run it. Open the windows? No way, burglars are in the streets. Anyway, the air outside is either hotter than inside or laden with pollutants.

Studies showed that the majority of heat wave fatalities occur in inner-city areas. The asphalt, brick and concrete jungle absorbs heat and retains it well into the night. On average, the inner city is 5 to 8°C hotter than the surrounding countryside—the heat island effect that NASA researched in 1998. Sensors in aircraft and satellites demonstrated that artificial surfaces reach temperatures 20–40°C higher than natural surfaces do—Salt Lake City rooftops, for instance, were 71°C. These figures also provide the answer: cities need more natural surfaces, especially trees, to cool down.

Unventilated apartment buildings and rooms without air conditioning can reach temperatures in excess of 50°C during heat wave conditions.

Even if ventilation is possible, the temperature drops to just above the outside air temperature. Since hot air rises, the top levels of apartment buildings suffer most. Insulation will keep the heat out for a day or two. But eventually the room succumbs to the environment and the insulation becomes a curse.

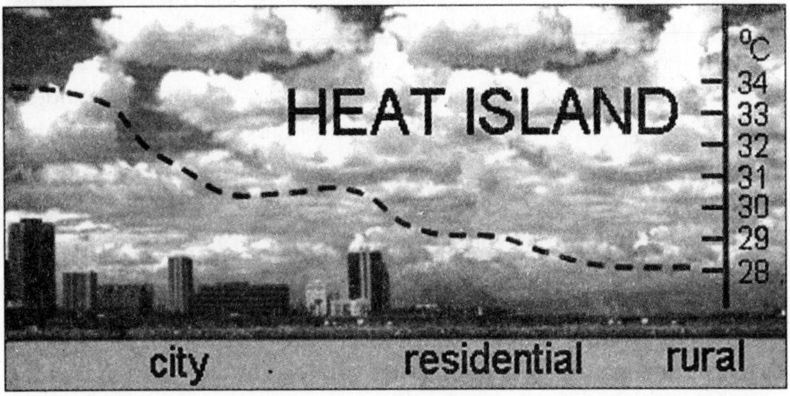

Now that we are aware of the heat island effects, we can modify building codes and include simple requirements to protect buildings from the heat, e.g. the inclusion of more natural areas. These will not only modify the climate but save electricity as well. A homeowner should consider the effects of extreme heat on the home.

You can try these simple measures to improve the climate of your home:

- Deciduous trees provide shade in the summer and let the sun's radiation heat the house in winter
- Orientate your home's rooms according to the elements; there is nothing worse than bedrooms facing the sun; it will virtually guarantee sleepless nights
- Include shaded verandas where possible
- Light-coloured walls and roofs will reflect some of the sun's radiation
- The eaves should be wide enough to shade the windows in summer.

Risk groups

The US Centres for Disease Control and Prevention published age-related mortality rates after the 1995 heat wave. The figures showed that

62% of the victims were 55 years or older. The elderly are less able to fend off the ill effects of extreme heat and some already suffer from underlying health problems and may take medication unsuitable for the heat. Many elderly citizens require extra care during heat wave periods. This care is often not available to people living alone or confined to bed due to physical and mental impairments. Air conditioning is either not present or not operating due to the high cost of electricity. Today local governments are making an effort to provide air conditioned shelters and/or subsidize the electricity cost.

Despite extensive warnings, children and pets are still left inside cars while the driver rushes into a store 'only for a second'. The seconds become minutes and the car reaches temperatures in excess of 65°C—unsustainable for life. The occupants can become seriously ill or die of heatstroke.

A large number of heat wave victims, however, are middle-aged and considered healthy. Strenuous outdoor activities, such as work or exercise, and excess alcohol or drugs can lead to dehydration and the collapse of the body's circulation or organs.

Most top athletes are aware of heat-related dangers and prepare accordingly. They religiously replace the lost fluids and electrolytes. They are fit and acclimatize before the competition. Of more concern are endurance sport events at a lower level of competition, such as at schools and local clubs. Unfortunately, many coaches are not aware of heat-related dangers or deliberately ignore them: the 'if you can't stand the heat then get out of the kitchen' attitude. The aim of any club event organizer or coach should be to avoid injury. They should take into consideration the severity of the weather condition and the fitness level of the athletes. Simply postponing an event or scheduling it for the cooler part of the day goes a long way in preventing injuries.

Beat the heat

On very cold days you put on your pullover. If this is not enough you add another layer of clothing, a parka or similar, or you wear thermal underwear. On hot days you obviously shed as many layers of clothes as possible. But once you reach the bare skin, or close to it, that is it. Other than moving into an air conditioned environment, you have to rely entirely on your body's ability to shed excess heat. The good news: you can help your body achieve this task.

- Avoid direct sunlight. Seek a shady spot wherever and whenever possible to give your temperature regulation system a chance to recover. A picnic in the shade of trees is better than a roasting on the beach.
- Schedule your exercises for the cooler parts of the day or avoid exercising altogether. Drink before, during and after exercises.
- If possible, stay in an air conditioned environment. If you don't have air conditioning, go to the movies or visit climate-controlled public places for a few hours. This is particularly true for the elderly and patients with heart or circulation problems.
- Aid the cooling effect of evaporation by using fans or moist towels. Take regular cool showers.
- Replenish the lost fluids and electrolytes. Drink plenty of water and remember to drink more than you 'feel' you should. Replace body salts with meals or drinks such as fruit juices or sport drinks. Persons on a fluid-restricted diet, however, should consult their physician before increasing the consumption.
- Avoid diuretic drinks such as alcohol, coffee and tea because they will increase your fluid loss. The icy-cold beer is only a temporary relief. Matters will get worse soon after the cold sensation stops.
- Outdoors, wear a wide-brimmed hat to provide shade and wear lightly coloured and loose-fitting clothes. Light colours reflect radiation. The difference between serious health damage and mild discomfort can be as simple as wearing the appropriate clothes.
- Acclimatize your body. If you are not used to hot conditions, start any strenuous activity slowly. Give yourself a few days rest when travelling to a hot climate.
- Sunscreen doesn't keep the heat away but it prevents sunburn. Sunburnt skin affects the cooling ability.
- Have small meals and more often. Avoid 'heavy' meals.
- Never leave kids or pets in the car on hot days.

Electric fans do nothing else than stir the air and this indirectly cools your body, as the air movement blows away the hot and moist layer near your skin. This allows more sweat to evaporate, thus cooling your body. If your skin were dry, you wouldn't feel a temperature difference. Consequently, if you want maximum cooling, keep your skin moist.

Fans are also useful at night to help exchange the air between a warm room and the hopefully cooler air outside.

Fans have their limits. When the temperatures soar towards 38°C or above, cooling becomes ineffective. The fan acts more like a hairdryer set on high heat. Your body's cooling mechanism is no longer capable of dealing with the hot air and your body temperature begins to rise. Now it is time for a cold shower instead.

Reacting to early warning signs prevents heat illnesses. Look out for signs such as dizziness, tiredness, profuse sweating, muscle cramps, rapid heartbeat, headache or nausea. If the intervals between toilet visits become longer and your urine is dark, you dehydrate. Not everyone is well equipped to recognize the signs, though. A lack of knowledge is the major hindrance. Health authorities often start their education campaigns when the hot weather has already arrived. Sadly, the arrival of a cool breeze may blow away any lessons learnt. Others recognize the signs but can't react due to physical restraints. Many frail and sick rely on help, which sometimes comes too late.

Employers are responsible for the welfare of their workers. Managers and supervisors need to know the symptoms of heat-related illnesses and should be aware of the state of health of their employees. As a precaution, they should reduce the work rate and increase the rest periods during heat wave conditions. Some employers are responsible enough and send their workers home when the temperatures at the work place exceed a certain limit.

Predicting heat waves is fairly easy. More often than not, the weather services issue warnings well in advance. The forecast includes an 'apparent' temperature that takes into account the expected humidity. A high temperature and low humidity is much more bearable than the same temperature is in combination with high humidity. The serious effects of a heat wave generally don't surface until the second or third day. This gives the authorities ample time to warn the public and take appropriate measures such as:

- Heat wave alerts on television, radio and in print media including public health information about the dangers of heat-related illnesses
- Home care providers educate their often frail patients during their visits
- Establishment of an information telephone line
- Advice to take care of relatives and friends without air conditioning

- Provision of air conditioned shelters in public places, such as shopping malls, libraries and churches
- Subsidized or free electricity for the poor during heat waves.

Chapter Five

Cold

Blame the cold for:

- Heart disorders
- Common cold
- Frostbite
- Chilblain
- Hypothermia

and more

Introduction

Have you managed to live through the hazards of the previous chapters unscathed? Don't become too complacent—this chapter may get you. Cold is responsible for more excess deaths and disorders than heat is. The higher figures aren't often apparent, however, as cold snaps don't have the same immediate impact as heat waves do. Cold-related illnesses manifest itself in much more subtle ways at first: kidneys produce more urine, hands and feet are constantly cold, or the blood pressure rises markedly. There are also the annual episodes of sneezing, wheezing and coughing. If the exposure to the cold persists, the ill effects lead to more serious problems such as frostbites or hypothermia.

We hear the amazing survival story of a child trapped under the ice of a frozen lake for one hour. A skier, lost and found in sub-zero temperatures, miraculously recovered in hospital after several hours of rewarming his frost-bitten body. Both were lucky? Probably. Despite the partly frozen condition of their 'shell' (skin, outer layers of fat and muscles), their core body temperatures were high enough to allow the survival of their essential organs. Most aren't so lucky: many soldiers who suffered from cold exposure during war have been left with body scars, or even developed painful symptoms decades later.

Human health is not the only casualty of cold weather, as wild, farm and domestic animals also suffer greatly. Newborn lambs and calves often don't survive an unseasonably cold outbreak. Some crops succumb to spring frosts, while fruit trees shed their flowers before they set fruit, leaving the farmer with a reduced or zero income. Substances expand in heat and contract in cold. The contractions of metal and concrete may become so severe that buildings suffer permanent damage. Your car suffers, too. The battery goes flat or the engine cracks if you push it too hard. Cold weather is the time to turn up the heater at home and at work. On such days, the energy consumption reaches peaks equally as high as during heat waves. The demand can be too high and blackouts occur.

Temperature Extremes

Vostok Station on Antarctica recorded the lowest temperature on Earth, –89°C. Obviously, exposure to such low temperatures is dangerous and explorers take appropriate precautions. Less dangerous, but of a much higher impact on the population's health, are the cold, wet and windy conditions of the temperate regions.

The body is cold or heat stressed when the temperature diverges excessively from the average. Melbourne, Australia is considered to have a temperate climate. Nevertheless, the temperatures can range from the highest recorded 45.6°C in summer to the lowest recorded of –2.8°C in winter. The US town of Warsaw, Missouri recorded extremes of 47.8°C as the highest and –40.0°C as the lowest.

Wind Chill

A breeze is very welcome in summer. The wind replaces the hot and humid air near your skin with cooler and drier air. More sweat can evaporate and cool your body. In winter you don't want this effect.

Lowest recorded temperatures

Continent	Temp. (deg C)	Temp. (deg F)	Place	Date
Antarctica	–89	–129	Vostok Station	21 Jul 1983
Asia	–68	–90	Oimekon, Russia	6 Feb 1933
N. America	–63	–81	Snag, Yukon, Canada	3 Feb 1947
Europe	–55	–67	Ust'Shchugor, Russia	unknown
S. America	–33	–27	Sarmiento, Argentina	1 Jun 1907
Africa	–24	–11	Ifrane, Morocco	11 Feb 1935
Australia	–22	–8	Charlotte Pass, N.S.W.	29 Jun 1994

You want the air near your skin to stay and provide a thin layer of insulation. In winter it is very important to wear clothes that limit the exchange of air near your skin—unless it is desired during exercise or outdoor work. A stormy winter's day, however, may penetrate whatever you are wearing and you will feel much colder than the actual air temperature around you.

Scientists incorporated the 'feel' factor into a wind chill index. For example, a measured temperature of 0°C feels like –16°C when a 37 km/h wind blows.

Wind chill – Celsius

	Air temperature									
	5	**0**	**–5**	**–10**	**–15**	**–20**	**–25**	**–30**	**–35**	**–40**
Wind km/h	Apparent temperature									
07	5	0	–5	–10	–15	–20	–25	–30	–35	–40
19	–3	–9	–16	–22	–28	–34	–41	–47	–53	–59
28	–6	–13	–21	–27	–34	–40	–48	–55	–61	–68
37	–8	–16	–24	–30	–37	–44	–52	–60	–66	–74
46	–10	–18	–26	–32	–39	–47	–55	–63	–70	–78
56	–11	–19	–28	–34	–41	–49	–57	–65	–73	–81
65	–12	–20	–29	–35	–42	–50	–58	–66	–74	–82
74	–12	–20	–29	–35	–42	–50	–58	–66	–74	–82

Cold and the body

Your teeth chatter, your body shivers and despite all efforts, you can't prevent it. The tiny hair on your body stand upright and try desperately to function as an insulating fur. Your skin looks bloodless and feels cold. All these reactions are an attempt by your body to preserve heat, although not a very successful one. Humans are well equipped to lose heat, but are less efficient in retaining it. Are we all meant to live on a tropical island?

Your body's reaction to heat loss is involuntary and driven by the hypothalamus, the tiny gland in the brain acting as a thermostat (see Chapter Four, 'Heat'). The hypothalamus is very sensitive to any temperature variation in your body. Even a small drop brings the temperature regulation mechanisms into action: blood vessels in the skin constrict to prevent excessive heat loss and muscles shiver to create heat.

The hypothalamus is a cruel gland, though. Its only concern is to keep the vital organs at an acceptable temperature, and eouldn't care less if your toes or fingers became icicles. All of the thermoregulation mechanisms are designed to protect the core. But if the system fails or becomes overwhelmed, cold-related illness or death is the consequence.

Every person reacts differently to thermal stress. Age, fitness level and underlying diseases play a major part in someone's reaction to cold.

The best way to get through a winter is to eat as much as you can, grow a thick winter coat, reduce your body temperature and find a hole in the ground where you can hibernate. Too easy for some animals, but not for us humans who don't acclimatize to the cold as well as we can to the heat. Nevertheless, repeated cold exposure does train the few defences to function more efficiently.

Since the body doesn't want to adjust to the cold very well, behavioural responses become the most important factors. Shelter and clothing protect from the cold. Eating high-energy food will increase the heat production, as will exercise—active muscles produce up to three-quarters of the total body heat, which stimulates the metabolism and further heat production. In fact, intense exercise and work can produce enough heat to maintain the desired body temperature under very cold conditions. Unfortunately, you can't sustain heavy physical activity for long periods and you will eventually lose heat.

Heat loss

To guarantee wellbeing, the body's core temperature needs to be maintained at around 36.9°C. What comprises the core? It includes all the vital organs such as heart, lungs, liver and kidneys 'central' to your body.

Response to core temperature drop

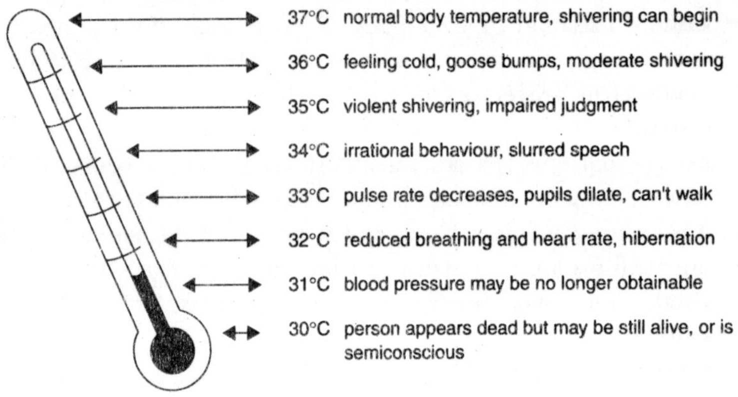

Because the brain is also important for your survival, it is part of the core—despite being nowhere near the centre.

Surrounding the core is the periphery. It includes the skin, the muscles, arms and legs. Shake the hands of someone on a cold day and you'll find out that the temperature of the periphery can be well below the core temperature—icy-cold hands. A cold periphery, however, is quite natural and, to a degree, an advantage. You constantly lose heat to a cooler environment until the periphery reaches the same temperature, and then the heat flow stops and you preserve heat. This has its limits. The problems begin when the surroundings have a very low temperature. In this case, the temperature exchange between your body and the environment doesn't stop and your core temperature starts to drop. Women have an advantage over men in that respect because their skin generally reaches a slightly lower temperature, so they have less heat to lose.

When you feel a chill, tiny muscles erect whatever is left of your body hair. 'Goose bumps' are a sign of this process. Obviously, this attempt to insulate the body is insufficient—you have to wear clothes. Scientists argue amongst themselves whether a layer of fat acts as insulator or not. So far, most agree that it does. People living in the cooler parts of the world have known this all along. They indulge in high-energy food during winter and leave the green salads for the summer.

As discussed previously, your body loses heat by conduction, convection, radiation and evaporation. Let's examine some of the aspects that relate to cold conditions:

- **Conduction.** Conduction is the transfer of heat from your body to a cooler substance by contact. 'Water and metal objects are excellent conductors of heat,' the scientist says. You wouldn't use the word 'excellent,' however, if you fell into an icy pond or have your skin frozen onto a metal object. Cold water absorbs your body's heat 25 times faster than air does, metal even faster. During cold conditions it is very important to remain dry. Just the sweat in your clothes after an exercise is sufficient to increase the rate of heat loss through conduction.
- **Convection.** If you stood naked in the snow, the warm air near your skin would slowly rise. You would lose heat by convection. Air is a good insulator, though. To be effective, your clothing has to keep a layer of warm air near the skin. Nose, ears, fingers and the face are usually uncovered and at the highest risk of developing cold injuries.
- **Radiation.** Your body doesn't have to be in contact with anything to lose heat. As long as you have some warmth left in your body, you will radiate and share your heat energy with things in your environment—including those people next to you. Unless you use your body warmth to give first aid to another person, you should be selfish and not share too much of your heat with other beings or things. The only substance you want to warm up by radiation is the material your clothing is made of—thus keeping the lost heat energy close to your skin. Some materials are even designed to reflect the heat energy back to your body, such as those used in space blankets.

The head, with its folds and cavities, is an efficient radiator of heat, which is desirable in the heat but not in the cold. Fortunately, evolution didn't push far enough to remove the remnant of protective fur from your head. Or has it?

- **Evaporation.** With every breath you exhale you lose heat energy. Some of the moisture in the lungs evaporates while breathing and is lost as water vapour when you exhale. The evaporation process requires energy—heat energy. This is fantastic when you want to get rid of some of your excess heat, but not so good if your body tries to survive the bitter cold. Exerting yourself in a cold environment leads to rapid breathing and to the cooling of your lungs and heart.

  Shovelling snow or any other strenuous exercise will make you sweat. This is OK as long as the water vapour can evaporate into the air through 'breathing' garments. If not, the sweat dampens your clothes and heat loss through conduction occurs.

Automatic temperature regulation

Shivering

Shivering is an involuntary muscle movement with the aim to create heat. With a strong will you can stop the action, but not for long. If you don't work your muscles, the body will do it for you. Extreme shivering can increase heat production by up to five times.

This bodily function does have its drawbacks. Muscle action requires fuel in the form of high-energy food. Without additional energy supply (eating), your body will soon be depleted of its reserves and become fatigued—now there's an excuse for some indulgence. Another negative effect of increased muscle activity is an increase in blood flow. More blood is diverted away from the core to the muscles, so heat loss is accelerated.

Metabolism

You can't survive on air and love alone. Even if you could, would you want to miss the pleasure of eating a chocolate cake topped with fresh strawberries? Oh no! Think of all those calories. They are good for something, though. They burn in the muscles, creating heat, and some of the excess deposits as an insulating layer of body fat.

Metabolism is the term for, among other things, the chemical process of digesting and absorbing food. When you eat (ingest) the cake, your stomach and intestines digest the delicious meal and create heat in the process. A good meal gives you a warm feeling in your belly. Absorbed nutrients are sent to the cells of all body parts, including the muscles, which then generate heat when they become active for a purpose or when they shiver involuntarily.

It is no coincidence that your core body temperature is ideal for the metabolic process. If the temperature drops, however, the chemical reaction slows down. To compensate for the drop, your metabolic rate increases slightly. Consequently, during cold conditions, the body requires more energy-rich food to support the body in its fight against the cold.

Vasoconstriction

Your skin is 'red hot' when the body needs to get rid of excess heat. On the other hand, your skin looks pale and feels cold when the body tries to preserve heat. The blood vessels in all the non-essential areas tighten (constrict) on command and limit the amount of hot blood that can reach the skin, thus preventing heat loss. The constriction can be so severe that almost no blood circulation exists in the non-essential body parts.

Your hands and feet are particularly vulnerable to this process. They may lose their agility and simple tasks, such as typing or opening a door with a key, become almost impossible. The cells in your muscles and skin, however, can't survive for long without some fresh blood supply. Occasionally the blood vessels will open up and allow some warm blood to reach the extremities. These pulses become less frequent and stop completely if the cold exposure continues.

Cold feet and cold hands are not necessarily a sign of poor blood circulation. It is the body's natural way of preserving heat. Acclimatized persons, and in particular women, manage this system quite well. Cold water immersion tests have revealed that skin temperatures of women were lower and the core temperatures remained higher than that of men.

Risk factors

Whether it is hot or cold, the elderly and, to some extent, the young are at a higher risk of developing cold-related illnesses and injuries. Nevertheless, certain factors predispose every person to heat loss and its consequences.

Some of the factors are:

- **Children.** The temperature control system in children and infants is not fully developed. This may delay the protective functions of shivering and vasoconstriction. The young have a large body surface relative to their weight. This allows more heat to escape during cold conditions. Children also tend to spend more time outdoors and are often ignorant of wet feet and hands.
- **Elderly.** The ability to sense temperature changes diminishes with age. The hypothalamus becomes sluggish and reacts slower to signals from the sensors. A lower metabolic rate and less physical activity creates less heat than may be necessary to sustain a healthy body temperature.
- Certain **medication and drugs** affect the body's ability to sense temperature changes and may impair judgment. Some prevent you from shivering, while others oppose blood vessel constriction. Many recreational drugs and nicotine, however, constrict blood vessels too much and limit or prevent short pulses of warm blood from reaching the extremities and the skin.
- **Diseases.** Various diseases, such as hormone disorders and diabetes, inhibit the function of the hypothalamus. They reduce the ability to sense and control body temperature. Some limit the blood flow within the vessels, while others decrease the metabolic rate and with it the ability to create heat. The heavy breathing and coughing of asthmatics results in excessive heat loss. A previous cold injury can make a person cold sensitive and more susceptible to further injury.
- **Alcohol** dilates the blood vessels and allows warm blood to reach the periphery. While this gives the person a temporary feeling of warmth and wellbeing, it has the eventual negative effect of heat loss at the core. It also delays the onset of shivering. Alcohol impairs judgment. An intoxicated person may not recognize the warning signs of a lurking cold injury.

- **Dehydration** reduces the volume of bodily fluids. Less fluid (blood) carries less heat into the periphery, therefore, increasing the danger of cold injuries to extremities.
- **Nutrition.** The body needs high-energy food to create heat and to sustain long periods of shivering or physical activity. Inadequate nutrition weakens the body's temperature control mechanisms.
- **Water.** A person immersed in cold water loses heat 25 times faster than he or she does in air of the same temperature. Even mild water temperatures are enough to cause hypothermia after a few hours. Wet or moist clothing also accelerates heat loss.
- **Cold objects and liquids.** Rapid conduction can cause skin to freeze to metal objects. Some liquids have a much lower freezing point than water has and may result in cold injuries if they get in contact with the skin.
- **Wind chill.** Air movement near the skin aids evaporation and cooling. Wind can drop the apparent temperature significantly.

COLD-RELATED DISORDERS

Cold diuresis

When you feel cold and have cold feet and hands do you have frequent toilet visits? Why? The body protects vital organs from cooling by reducing the blood flow to the outer layers of the body. More warm blood is kept in and around the body's core, increasing the volume and pressure at the same time. Unfortunately, the brain may perceive this as an unnecessary increase. It instructs the kidneys to extract some of the fluids from the blood and shed it as urine.

Once the reason for the cold is eliminated, the blood flows back to the periphery. All these toilet trips, however, reduced fluid levels considerably and the body may experience mild dehydration.

Heart and circulatory diseases

The relationship between weather extremes and mortality rates is well documented. Extreme heat or cold increases the number of heart attacks dramatically. Just a moderate drop of 10°C in temperature raises the risk by 13% in the population of middle-aged French men. Winter is the season for heart attacks amongst all sexes and age groups in the US, with 53% more cases than during summer.

Data collected from patients fitted with heart rhythm regulators (defibrillators) gave some proof of the relationship between weather extremes and heart diseases. When scientists compared the result with climatic data obtained form the national weather service, they found that heart rhythm abnormalities are more frequent on days with either very high or very low outside air temperatures. Some patients reacted immediately to temperature changes, others' reactions were delayed by 2–3 days.

While there is no more doubt that cold weather increases the risk of heart or circulatory disease, the question remained whether the link is only present in cold climate regions. Not so; 'cold' is relative. The mortality rate during Hawaii's winter increases by 22%, a figure similar to some cold climate regions.

Why do the heart and the circulation react so violently to temperature drops? There is no single answer. Cold and wet weather is the time of semi-hibernation and indulgence. Unhealthy eating habits and less activity contribute to an increase in heart diseases, but aren't the only reasons. You can blame the weather for physical changes to your blood.

Previously you read that the body reacts to cold by constricting the blood vessels in the periphery of your body. The heart has to work harder to squeeze blood through the narrow vessels. This may be too much for a sick heart. Surveys of blood donors revealed that blood pressure rose significantly after temperature drops. Published figures showed increases of between 12 and 18 mmHg. While such an increase is not significant for a healthy person, it is sometimes a deciding factor for a person suffering already from high blood pressure. Medical practitioners should take the seasonal effect into account when treating hypertension.

Blood and the cold

- Increased blood pressure
- Lower blood volume
- Higher cholesterol level
- Increased viscosity
- Higher risk of blood clotting

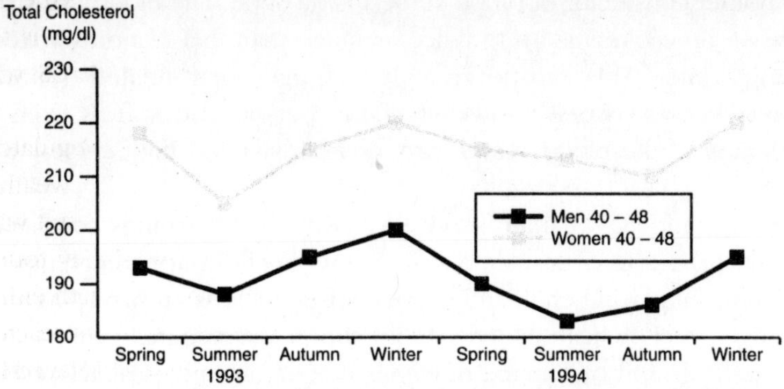

Arzte Zeitung 1999 (German Magazine for General Practitioners)

Lower temperatures also change the composition of the blood. The change is almost immediate and persists for up to two days. The number of particles in the blood, such as platelets, red blood cells, fibrinogen and cholesterol, increases in cold conditions and make the blood thicker (increased viscosity). Some tests showed an increase in viscosity by up to 21%. The risk of blood clotting increases also and, together with the high viscosity, may lead to blocked blood vessels in the heart, brain or lungs.

If this is not enough to make you sick, add a little overexertion. Any physical activity is good for your body, but in moderation. Slow down if you suspect or know of problems with your heart or circulation. Shovelling snow off your footpath, or any other strenuous activity, together with the cold effect on your body, can be a lethal combination. Hospital emergency departments register a significant increase of patient numbers after heavy snowfall.

People with a history of heart attacks have a higher risk of reacting negatively to the cold than those with no previous heart troubles have, some for 2 to 10 years after an attack. More women than men are burdened with extreme weather sensitivity after a heart attack.

Cold weather is also the time of cold and flu medicines. Some can exaggerate the cold effect. Decongestants, for example, work by constricting enlarged blood vessels in your nose. Unfortunately, they may do the same to the rest of your body's vessels and raise the blood pressure. Most medications carry warnings. If in doubt, ask your doctor.

Another constrictor of blood vessels is nicotine. The blood pressure increase of smokers is up to twice as much than that of non-smokers during winter. This can be enough to trigger heart-related trouble. Matters become worse, however, if the person also suffers from a hardening of the blood vessels (arteriosclerosis) and high cholesterol levels.

Some national weather services incorporate warnings for heart patients in their forecasts. Meteorologists warn of low apparent temperatures, such as wind chill, and of weather conditions known to have a negative effect on heart patients. Heart clinics can prepare by informing their patients and by limiting therapies that involve physical activities.

Allergy to cold

Many, if not most people, dislike the cold weather. For some, however, it is not a matter of choice—they become physically sick. Cold urticaria is an allergy to cold, characterized by localized red swollen marks on the skin. These wheals can vary in size and are often accompanied by itching pain. The allergy may even appear in summer when the person swims in cold water and can lead to drowning if the airways are narrowed by the swellings.

Common cold and influenza

Fellow travellers on the train cough and sneeze behind their newspapers. At the office, the first empty chairs forewarn of the start of a flu epidemic. Yes, it is winter—the season of coughs, wheezes and sniffs, of common cold and influenza.

Historians describe several devastating influenza epidemics. An estimated 20 million people lost their lives during the 'Spanish flu' in 1918. Since then, medical advances contained major outbreaks so that today 'only' thousands become victims. The US experienced an epidemic in 1957 that killed an estimated 70,000 people, followed by another outbreak in 1968 with 34,000 victims.

Approximately 200 different kinds of viruses cause symptoms of the common cold. Several others lead to influenza. Often, the first signs are sneezing and a sore throat, followed by the inflammation of the sinuses (sinusitis) and the lungs (bronchitis). Fever generally occurs with influenza only. A third kind of virus (Herpes simplex) attacks the weakened body and causes a cold sore.

These illnesses are most frequent during the colder months of the year. However, the lower temperatures alone have nothing to do with the increase in frequency. Just the opposite: viruses and bacteria multiply more readily at milder temperatures. You can't catch a cold or influenza because the thermometer has plummeted.

The lower temperatures are an indirect cause, though. Whenever the person next to you sneezes or coughs, he or she dislodges tiny droplets that contain a large number of viruses. In summer, the fresh air outdoors rapidly dilutes the density of the viruses and the risk of catching the germ is lower—not so in winter. During the winter months people tend to spend more time indoors with the windows closed to save energy. The virus concentration is high, and with it comes the risk of inhaling a few. Winter's low level of ultraviolet sunlight also plays a part. Sufficient ultraviolet rays during the summer period help kill the viruses.

Continually changing weather conditions stress the body and weaken the immune system. Viruses and bacteria find ways to get past the defence system. A runny nose, however, is a sign that at least part of the system is working. It is a healthy body reaction to get rid of the intruders. So, don't stop this reaction by using nasal sprays. Use a handkerchief instead.

With every exposure to any of the viruses' strains, the body develops immunity and protects the person against that particular germ when it appears the next time. The children's immune system, however, hasn't had much experience with viruses. It is still learning how to recognize the different strains. Until their body develops the relevant immunities, they will be sick more often. Vaccines induce the body to produce such immunities.

Diabetes

The climatic effect on diabetes is to date not well researched. Scientists have no doubt that seasonal patterns exist, but are unsure of any short-term influences. So far, statistics show that insulin-dependent diabetes mellitus (IDDM) has its beginnings more often in winter than in other seasons. Some reports suggest that lower temperatures increase the level of glycosylated haemoglobin, a substance that results from blood sugar attaching itself to gas-carrying red blood cells (haemoglobin). A seasonal change in eating and exercise habits, however, may have a greater negative effect on diabetes sufferers.

Winter asthma

The indoor lifestyle during cold conditions is one cause of aggravated asthma. The room is often filled with airborne allergens such as dust mites, smoke particles from wood fires, pet hair and viruses. Fresh air will dilute the particles and relieve the symptoms. But cold dry air can make matters worse. The airways tend to narrow and the mucus lining thickens, making breathing more difficult. Asthmatic children in particular display more symptoms during outdoor activities. Breathing through a scarf around the mouth is often enough to pre-warm the air.

Raynaud's disease

Named after a French physician, the disease is a disorder that affects the blood vessels in extremities such as fingers, toes, ears, lips and nose. The vessels constrict spasmodically, thereby interrupting the blood flow to the relevant body part. In extreme cases, the blood flow almost stops. This can cause the death and decay of body tissue (gangrene).

Chances are you either suffer from this disease yourself or you have experienced the icy handshake of an affected person. According to a recent US survey, approximately 5–10% of the population suffer to some degree from Raynaud's disease. Figures supplied from outside the US are somewhat lower. There is no argument, however, that women between the ages of 15 and 40 comprise the majority of diagnosed cases—three times as many as in the male population. The disease is not limited to regions with cold climates. While there are fewer people affected in milder climates, those who are affected experience more attacks when the weather turns cold.

Low temperatures and emotional stress are common triggers of Raynaud's disease. But it can also manifest itself as a secondary symptom to skin disorders such as lupus and sceloderma. Some users of vibratory tools, such as pneumatic hammers and chain saws, can develop the disease—especially when the tools are handled in cold conditions.

The constriction of blood vessels is a natural protection against the cold. The system in patients with Raynaud's disease, however, is too sensitive and constrictions are too intense. Severe constriction of the small arteries causes a collapse of blood circulation in the affected body part. As a consequence, the limbs undergo unwanted physical changes.

The first obvious reaction is a waxy-looking skin. If the attack continues, the lack of oxygen in the tissue turns the skin blue and the patient experiences a tingling sensation and painful throbbing. Such an attack can last for several hours. Finally, the condition fades and blood will flow back into the arteries, causing a reddening of the skin. The disease can progress further, resulting in a prolonged or permanent interruption of the blood flow. The affected body parts, most notably the fingers, become permanently thin and shiny white. To make matters worse, nicotine and certain drugs or medication constrict blood vessels further, intensifying the symptoms.

Doctors generally recommend self-help measures, such as keeping the affected body parts warm to prevent tissue damage. They recommend quitting smoking, controlling stress and exercising regularly. There is also medication available to relax the small blood vessels in the periphery.

Accidents

You can hear your neighbour swear at the weather when he or she slips on the doorstep, twisting an ankle in the process. Cold-weather clothing also often contributes to accidents as they're usually heavy, cumbersome and restrict movement. Hoods and hats limit your peripheral vision and muffle noise. Also, performing awkward jobs with thick gloves is certainly not easy.

Winter hazards cause injuries and death. The US National Hazard Statistics of 1997 lists 84 fatalities and 573 injuries as being caused by winter storms and 6 fatalities and 43 injuries by ice.

Carbon monoxide (CO) is a silent killer. The odourless and invisible gas is a result of incomplete combustion in slow-burning fires and idling vehicles. What has this to do with blaming the weather? A lot really. You don't heat your house in summer, do you? Every year, many people with open fires become ill with headache, dizziness and drowsiness. If victims don't notice these symptoms due to their drowsiness, they may become unconscious and die.

Similarly to CO poisoning, burns are an indirect result of cold weather conditions. People, in particular children, get burnt from touching hot surfaces of stoves and open fireplaces. Others get injured or die in a house fire that originated with the good intention of drying a wet towel in front of a heater.

Chilblain

Your extremities are about to suffer again. Chilblain is an inflammatory swelling to the skin of your feet, hands, face and ears, caused by cold exposure. In contrast to frostbite, the skin does not freeze, but may leave some permanent damage to the fine blood vessels. In instances where the affected areas become sensitive to cold, the symptoms return quickly after every exposure. The skin develops red pimples or patches and may itch, burn or sting. It can worsen to painful swellings and blisters. The preferred treatment is to gradually warm the affected area, as sudden rewarming aggravates the condition.

Frostnip

An untreated chilblain may develop into frostnip. Frostnip freezes the outer layers of fingers, toes, face and ears. Other than exposure to severe cold, contact with cold metal or liquid is often the cause. Poor circulation in the extremities worsens the situation. If treated immediately, the injury is generally reversible. If not, the condition develops further into the dangerous frostbite.

Frostnip is hard to distinguish from frostbite. The frozen layer of the skin appears similarly white and waxy, but feels rubbery. In contrast, frost-bitten flesh is hard as deeper layers are frozen. The nipped skin turns red and sometimes painfully swollen after rewarming. Like sunburn, the affected area sheds a dead layer of skin after a few days of healing. Repeated frostnip injury may lead to cold sensitivity.

As with chilblains, preventing cold exposure by wearing the appropriate clothing is better than a painful cure. If you do have to be in the elements, always check your exposed skin for numbness and look out for a change in colour. Gently warm nipped areas. Do not massage the area because the ice crystals can damage the skin tissue, aggravating the injury.

Frostbite

Skin and flesh freezes at about –2°C. Superficial frostnip heals, but the freezing of deeper layers results in permanent damage. Circulation stops, fine arteries burst, blood clots and cells die. Mechanical damage occurs when the ice crystals puncture cells during rubbing of the area or if the person continues to walk on affected feet. The dead tissue will eventually decompose and, depending on the severity of the damage, the limb may have to be amputated.

Sounds terrible? It is quite fortunate, really. Because that is how the temperature regulator, the hypothalamus, reacts to cold extremes. Its loyalty is towards the essential organs to keep you alive—a hand or foot can be discarded. Frostbite is, therefore, not life-threatening. But it leaves the victim with scars and long-term complications such as persistent pain, joint problems and an increased cold sensitivity.

Over 3,000 male conscripts of the Finnish defence force took part in a study to find the number of incidences and severity of frostbites. The researchers found that almost 2 per 1,000 conscripts developed frostbites annually. The majority of injuries were superficial and common to the ear (58%). Most at risk were those not wearing the appropriate clothing, such as earflaps or scarves. Individual cold sensitivity was a significant factor.

Frostbites are caused by:

- **Low temperatures.** Temperatures below –2°C can induce frostbites on exposed body parts. The danger increases when low temperatures combine with **moisture** (wet clothing) and **wind chill**.
- **Supercooled substances.** Metal reaches temperatures well below freezing point. Skin and flesh freeze instantly when in contact.

- **Tight-fitting garments** such as shoes, hats, watchbands and belts restrict the blood flow and increase the likelihood of cold injuries.
- **Medication and drugs.** Some substances, e.g. nicotine, constrict the blood vessels in the periphery.

Frostbitten skin appears waxy-white and is rigid. An initial tingling sensation and feeling of coldness soon gives way to numbness. Due to the lack of pain, the victim may no longer be aware of the injury. A superficial frostbite contains some life in the tissue and thawing results in swelling and blistering of the area. Frostbites, which involve freezing of the muscles and/or bones, don't show signs of blistering after rewarming. The exception is the area bordering the frostbite, which has superficial damage where blood-filled blisters may develop.

Prevention is the same as for frostnip. Treating frostbite is a gentle process. The old theory of rubbing the affected area with snow is no longer applicable, as it will further damage the tissue. Obtain emergency medical assistance as quickly as possible.

Trench foot and immersion foot

If only your unhappy potted daisy could talk. Unhappy because it has to grow in a prison pot; and unhappy because the well-meant caring is often overdone by too much watering. The poor daisy is wilting. The roots are rotting.

Soldiers aren't daisies but their plight may also go unheard by their carers. Hundreds of thousands of Napoleon's and Hitler's soldiers walked through mud and slush in their quest to conquer Russia. The adversaries of WWI spent days, weeks and months in soggy French trenches. Like the daisy's roots, human feet don't appreciate wet conditions. Add low temperatures and feet will rot—literally.

Trench foot has its name from the disease that debilitated WWI soldiers during trench warfare in wet and cold conditions. In spite of its association with the military, equally at risk are outdoor workers, hunters, hikers and anglers. They often wear tight-fitting and non-breathing rubberized boots over a lengthy period. Immersion foot is similar but, as the name suggests, is associated with continuous immersion of feet in water.

Although trench foot and immersion foot are non-freezing injuries, the symptoms compare with those of frostbite. They are localized and occur mostly, but not exclusively, at the feet. At first, the affected area underneath the soft skin itches, tingles and feels numb. Later, red or blue blisters appear that either weep or bleed. The treatment for trench foot is similar to frostbite.

Hypothermia

A pity that you can't behave like other warm-blooded creatures and feast on the delicious autumn offerings, then slumber through the cold and wet season. Wouldn't this be great—unless you're a diehard winter sports fanatic. Hibernating animals can drop their body temperature sufficiently to slow all their body organ activity, thus reducing their metabolism to a minimum. For a human, however, such a temperature drop can be fatal. Perhaps we are meant to live on tropical islands after all, where food is plentiful all year round—a nice dream.

But dreaming can be the first sign of hypothermia. A drop in body temperature affects your ability to think clearly and, as for a hibernating animal, slows your body functions. This makes hypothermia particular dangerous, especially if the effect is combined with alcohol or other drug intoxication. Many revellers quite happily lie down in the snow for a snooze and never wake up again.

If you fall into a fire, you are made aware of the change in temperature very quickly. Hypothermia, on the other hand, can sneak up on you. The elderly and very young can die in their sleep in cold bedrooms: the latter's sense of the cold hasn't yet developed and the former has lost theirs. The cause of death is often attributed to various different reasons because underlying health problems and/or drug effects can mask the real culprit.

The signs and symptoms are difficult to recognize because the victim initially behaves as if under the influence of alcohol or drugs: irrational behaviour, confusion, loss of coordination and slurred speech are some of the signs. When hypothermia progresses, the victim becomes unconscious and may not show any obvious heartbeat or pulse. Breathing is very faint. Despite appearing almost dead, most people survive with appropriate treatment. Permanent damage is likely, though, if the core temperature drops below 26.5°C. Hypothermia is a medical emergency, and is as common in summer as it is in winter.

Healthy people are actually more at risk from accidental hypothermia. Exposure to the elements during outdoor activities, such as work, commuting or travel, poses a risk. Cold water particularly drains body heat quickly—the unlucky passengers of the *Titanic*, immersed in icy water, probably lost consciousness within 15 minutes. Even relatively mild water of 20°C will drain body heat within a few hours and unconsciousness will set in. Wet clothing has the same effect, although it will take longer.

Hypothermia is defined as a drop in the body's core temperature to a level that impairs normal body functions, and three stages are recognized. Mild hypothermia occurs at a core temperature above 35°C, severe when it drops below 32°C, with moderate hypothermia in-between. Controlled hypothermia is commonly used in neurosurgery and cardiac bypass surgery to slow the functions and oxygen requirements of organs.

The term *afterdrop* is sometimes mentioned in connection with hypothermia. It occurs during rewarming of the body when the blood vessels in the periphery expand, allowing blood from the warmer core to mix with the still cooler blood of the outer layers. The cool mixture then circulates back to the body's centre and causes another temperature drop.

COLD WEATHER MORTALITY

If main events of our lives were marked on a perpetual calendar that we could glimpse at will, then the odds are up by 10–15% that we find the date for our last heartbeat marked on a day in the colder season. We may never be able to cheat death, but with the right knowledge, we may be able to advance its date by a few years.

Humans are, well, only human and differ in their reasoning, statisticians especially so. What is included in cold weather mortality rates? Thousands may die during worldwide influenza epidemics, but can their deaths be directly linked to the aggravating effects of cold weather? Probably not. Someone gets lost on a skiing trip and dies of hypothermia. Is he or she part of the cold weather mortality rate? Most likely yes. The US directly attributes between 100 and 800 deaths a year to cold, depending on who issues the figures.

The guidelines on what constitutes a direct cause differ between countries and often between states. What is clear, however, is that the total number of deaths, directly and indirectly linked to the cold, increases significantly during a prolonged temperature drop below the average. The US numbers increased by more than 5,000 during a cold spell in 1983. Of course, the temperature average is relative to a region and people in a temperate climate suffer at much milder temperatures than those living in colder regions.

The Eurowinter Group highlights the regional differences. For each degree below 18°C, the mortality rate increased by 2.15% in Athens, but only by 0.27% in Finland. Once the temperature reaches 0°C or less, however, the mortality rate in Finland does rise significantly as well. In Yekaterinenburg, Russia, for example, the rate increases by 1.15% for every one degree drop below the freezing point.

The good news is that there's a slow decline in the rate of excess mortality during cold weather. Citizens of wealthy nations can afford well-insulated housing and efficient heating systems. Nevertheless, for those days when it breaks down or you're out of doors, you need to be aware of the ill effects of cold on your body.

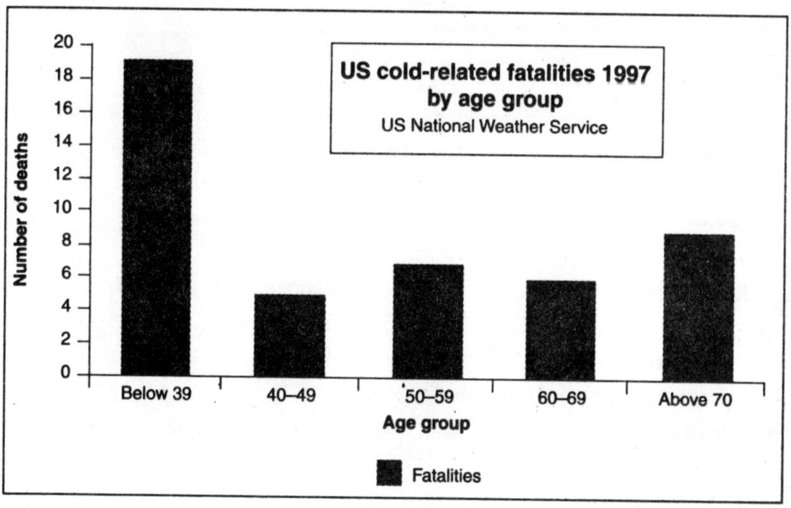

BEAT THE COLD

Follow the swallows to warmer regions. The thought isn't too far-fetched—many retirees are almost as predictable as swallows in their migratory behaviour. Every autumn, caravans and mobile homes clog the major roads leading to the sunnier locales, their passengers searching for warmth to soothe their aching bodies. By the time early summer arrives and the temperatures rise too high, these migratory people return to the cooler regions.

Avoiding the cold is obviously the best prevention, but not always practical. Life has to go on and work has to be done—but safely. The less time you are exposed to the cold the less chance you have of being injured or getting ill. But try to explain this to the kids up bright and early after the first snowfall. They must build that snowman. They must throw snowballs at their friends. They must cover themselves from head to toes in snow. The snow may be slushy but that won't deter them. 'Hey kids, that's enough. You are getting cold,' the concerned parent shouts. 'Oh no. We are warm. Honestly,' comes the stuttered reply from a shivering pair of blue lips.

Awareness is just as important as avoidance. Know the cold injury symptoms and first aid treatments. Be aware of the weather forecast and wind chill. Be prepared.

Clothing

Instead of wearing a super-thick ski jacket above your shirt, you should consider wearing multiple layers of loose-fitting clothing. This way, you can remove or add layers if you feel too hot or cold. The trapped air between each layer and in the padding of a garment acts as perfect insulation.

The outer layer should preferably be waterproof and windproof. But this is a trade-off between the need for protection against the environment and the need for ventilation. A waterproof outer layer acts like a sauna suit because your sweat can't evaporate, and collects in the clothing. Any initial feeling of warmth soon gives way to cold. Such a garment works best while outdoors when you stand or sit and you don't sweat much, but is useless when you work or exercise hard. Dirt or sweat, however, clogs the space between the padding fibres and leave less room for insulating warm air. On the other hand, a loosely knitted jumper allows the wind to penetrate deep into the clothing and carry away the warm layer of air. Tightly knit fabrics or modern microfibres that repel or resist rainwater but allow 'breathing' are a compromise.

You lose a large amount of heat if your head is exposed to the cold. More than half of total heat loss can occur from the head. Unless you are too hot and need to radiate heat, wear a hat, cap or hood, preferably with ear protection. A scarf, facemask or balaclava protects the skin on your face. Just take it off, though, when you enter a bank!

Mittens provide a larger volume of insulating air for your fingers. Gloves, however, win the contest when you have to perform an awkward task, such as opening a zipper in a hurry.

Clean, dry and thick socks warm your feet; a rubber sole on your shoes protect from moisture; and a permeable material for the upper part of the shoe provides ventilation. Your feet will thank you with the loveliest fragrance they ever produced. Rubber boots, however, prevent ventilation. If worn too long, trench foot or immersion foot develops. Tight shoes restrict blood circulation and add to the risk of cold injury.

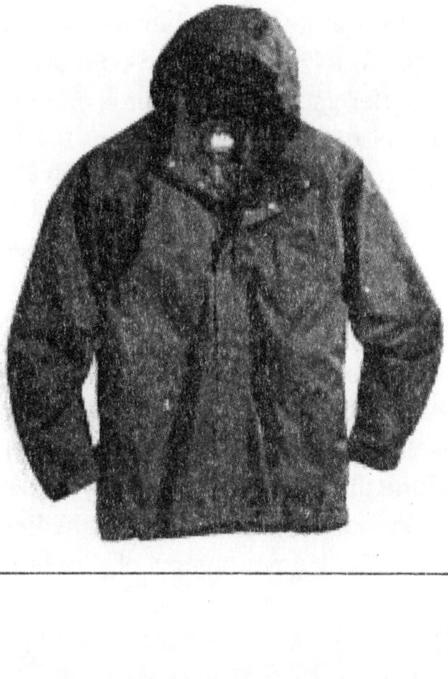

The ideal winter clothing:

- absorbs sweat
- deflects the wind
- is lightweight
- is waterproof
- is warm
- is durable
- insulates
- ventilates
- is easy to wear and remove

Your body

Healthy people often ignore the first signs and symptoms of a cold-related injury or illness: 'A little cold won't kill me,' they say. They are correct, but the emphasis is on 'little'. On the other hand, children and the elderly may not be aware of the early warning signs. You, as an informed person, should watch for signs and symptoms, such as persistent shivering, from yourself and others.

Having cold hands and feet is bad enough, but add moisture and the feeling of cold can turn to injury. The heat loss increases dramatically if a part of your body is moist or wet and exposed to the air, in particular moving air. Your fingers can become so stiff that simple manual tasks are impossible. Keep feet, hands and exposed skin dry.

Prevent conductive heat loss as much as possible. If you have to sit on cold ground, place some insulating material between your backside and the ground, so you don't lose heat to it, and don't touch anything metal either, as it can reach even lower temperatures and can freeze your skin instantly. Avoid substances that constrict blood vessels, such as nicotine and certain medication. Talk to your doctor if you are cold sensitive.

Be active without overexerting yourself. The combination of cold weather and intense physical activity could be too much for patients with heart or circulatory trouble. Just breathing cold air may be sufficient to lower the body temperature below the danger level. Wear a scarf or similar in front of your mouth to pre-warm the cold air. This is particular important for asthma sufferers, as cold dry air is one of the recognized asthma triggers. If all else fails, move indoors for your exercises.

Your house

Prepare your house for the winter by installing or improving insulation. Don't forget to cover exposed water pipes if you expect temperatures below freezing. Keep steps and walkways free of ice to prevent slipping. Have your heating checked before the cold season starts, as partly blocked exhausts can lead to carbon monoxide poisoning. Is the heater adequate for the size of your home? Many governments of places with cold climates provide financial support for their low-income citizens to either insulate their homes or to supplement energy costs.

Remember that even relatively mild temperatures can cause hypothermia if a person is exposed to the elements for some time. An easy-to-read thermometer for the bedroom of your elderly relative could be a life-saving birthday present. Institutions such as old people's homes or homes for the mentally disadvantaged have to be especially prepared, as their patients' responses to the cold may be ineffective.

Outdoor work

Someone has to brave the bitter cold and fix those broken power lines, so others can earn their income in the comfort of heated office buildings. Someone has to work the oil rigs in gales and storms so that others can drive their cars to work. If appalling weather isn't bad enough, cumbersome cold-weather clothing and slippery surfaces add further to the strain of outdoor work.

Under such conditions, how can workers keep up their morale? Perhaps they visualize a hot Irish stew. Workers need high-energy food. Their caloric requirement in the cold is up to 50% higher than it is under warm conditions.

Workers should be trained to perform tasks while wearing cold-weather clothing, as it's not only cumbersome, but sometimes hazardous. Hats and hoods restrict peripheral vision, thus compromising safety. Glasses and goggles frequently fog over, reducing visibility; while the loose end of a scarf or belt can get caught in machinery and cause injury. Conventional switches and buttons are difficult to operate with gloves or mittens, so the employer should ensure that the workplace or machinery is designed for cold weather operations.

The properties of substances change with temperature: flexible material can become hard and brittle, and even the metal teeth on zippers can freeze or break in extreme conditions. The good intention of taking cold metal tools to a warm environment will make the air's water vapour condense and may cause corrosion in the possibly very expensive object.

Chapter Six

Sun

Blame the sun for:

- Sunburn
- Aged skin
- Light sensitivity
- Non-cancerous growth
- Cancer
- Snow blindness
- Cataracts
- Immune system disorders and more

Introduction

The sun brings warmth, light and life—so it's often been thought of as a god. Ancient cultures worshipped the sun, offering food and even human sacrifices in religious ceremonies to keep the god happy. Most of the time the deity obliged and regularly drove across the sky in his or her golden chariot. Our ancestors, however, could be quite naughty at times. At quite regular intervals, when the fruit and vegetables or attractive young human just weren't good enough, the god turned black in anger, was eclipsed or darkened the sky.

Not much has changed since then. Today, millions of people worship the sun—especially during school holidays. They flock to the beaches and stay at the foreshore temples. In the morning they pray for sunshine and curse every tiny cloud. They lay out their near-naked bodies on top of ceremonial towels and offer their health and sometimes their lives to the sun. In return, the sun turns white skin to bronze and presents everybody with a free dose of vitamin D.

Who is this sun god? It is a giant ball of glowing hydrogen and helium, ignited just under 5 billion years ago. By the way, the word 'helium' comes from the Greek word *helios* and stands for 'sun.' The earth just happens to circle the sun at a safe distance to avoid the scorching heat, but close enough to deny any frost permanent residency in most of the earth's regions. The glowing gases of the sun reach temperatures of around 5,500°C at the surface—certainly an efficient space heater for your family room and no gas bills for another 5 billion years. Of course it wouldn't fit: being 1,392,000 km in diameter, the sun is about 109 times the size of the earth.

The sun's heat also drives the weather. The rays heat a variety of the earth's surfaces to different temperatures and also the air above. The air over a warm patch rises and leaves an area of low pressure near the surface. Cooler air from the relatively high pressure in the neighbourhood eventually replaces the risen air and fills the low. The action of replacement, whether small scale or global, is the wind, while the border between the cooler and warmer air is called a front. The sun's heat also evaporates water. The wind carries the water vapour into the atmosphere where it may condense and create clouds or rain.

Visible sunlight is the first thing you notice when the sun rises. The warmth of the infrared rays is probably next. But these are not the only components of electromagnetic waves originating from the sun. The known forms include rays with very short wavelengths, such as gamma rays and X-rays. At the same time, the sun sends out slightly longer waves in the visible and non-visible light range: ultraviolet, visible and infrared light. The spectrum also includes microwaves, radio waves, electric and long waves.

Visible sunlight

Colour is perception. The green traffic light is only green because you were told as a child that the colour you see is green. *The Lady in Red* looks absolutely gorgeous in her red dress. Does she? Many people have colour blindness and aren't aware of it. To them the red dress is just another shade of grey.

Visible light is nothing other than a package of electromagnetic waves with very short wavelengths of between 400 and 700 nanometres (1 nm = 10^{-9} metre). When the eyes receive the whole package, you see it as white light. Sometimes substances break the package and send the waves individually to your eyes. Raindrops do so when the sun is at a certain angle, and break the light into the colours of the rainbow.

The fabric of the red dress reflects only the longer wavelengths of the light: around 700 nm. A violet-coloured dress reflects light with the shortest visible wavelengths: approximately 400 nm. All other colours are at wavelengths in-between. To be thoroughly accurate, you may as well rename the previously mentioned song title to *The Lady Wearing a Dress Reflecting Light with a Wavelength of 700 nm.*

With the exception of deep-sea and underground creatures or plants, most life forms depend on the visible light in some form or another. Light gives you the chance to enjoy your surroundings. It gives you vision. But light is also a life clock that controls the day and night cycle in plants, animals and humans. It reminds you when to wake and sleep (circadian rhythm). The level of light intensity sensed by your eyes affects the amount of melatonin released by the pineal gland. Melatonin is a hormone thought to influence the circadian rhythm. Jet lag and sleep disorders are the consequences when this rhythm is out of sync.

Plants, animals and humans detect seasonal changes in light intensity. Light activates the need to breed, hibernate or migrate in some animals. It triggers plant seeds to germinate and flowers to open. Shorter daylight hours bring about the 'winter blues' in some people and may even develop into serious depressions (Seasonal Affective Disorder, or SAD).

Scientists are now assessing whether the present artificial lighting in homes, offices, schools etc. is impacting negatively on our performance, mood and health. They argue and test the possibility that humans require the whole spectrum of light to function properly. Most modern artificial light sources radiate only part of the spectrum.

Arguably the most important function of light is to provide food. You need sunlight in order to have your evening meal—not to find the steak or carrot on your plate, but to have the food there in the first place. The plants draw water from the ground and store it in their leaves. The light energy splits the water molecules into hydrogen and oxygen atoms. Hydrogen then combines with carbon dioxide to create a form of sugar. The leftover oxygen is released into the atmosphere for your benefit. By this chemical process, called photosynthesis, the plant becomes either a direct food source for you in the form of fruit or vegetables; or is an indirect food source in the form of meat, milk or egg from the animal that beat you to the lettuce.

Ultraviolet radiation

You marvel at the beauty of a butterfly's wings. To you the pattern of the left wing is identical to the wing on the right. But what you see is *not* what you get—seen under ultraviolet light, the pattern of each wing is very different. If you had the facetted eyes of a butterfly you too could see light with shorter wavelengths than that of violet light (400 nm). You would see the world with different eyes—metaphorically and literally.

UV light radiates at wavelengths between 100 and 400 nm. Whereas visible light is broken up into its primary colours of red, green and blue and many shades, UV light has less fancy names for its subdivision: UVA, UVB, and UVC.

Ultraviolet light				**Visible light**						
Colour	UVC	UVB	UVA	Violet	Blue	Cyan	Green	Yellow	Orange	Red
Wavelength (nm)	100–280	280–320	320–400	400	450	500	550	580	600	700

UVC has the shortest wavelengths. It is absorbed by the atmosphere and doesn't reach the earth's surface. The amount of UVB radiation reaching the ground depends largely on the state of the ozone layer in the upper atmosphere, which we all know is thinning. Record levels of UVB radiation have been recorded in parts of Europe, North America and Australasia. UVA, on the other hand, radiates at longer wavelengths and reaches the earth's surface almost unhindered, as it is not absorbed by the ozone layer.

While the sun is the major source of UV radiation, some man-made sources also produce high levels of UV light. Tanning devices, such as sun beds and sun lamps, emit mostly UVA, but some radiate UVB as well. The processes of arc welding and sterilization of medical equipment produce UV radiation. The white light of quartz halogen lamps is becoming increasingly popular at work and at home, but unshielded globes expose you to harmful UV radiation, especially at close quarters.

How much radiation you will absorb depends on many factors:

- The **angle** at which the UV rays strike your body or the earth's surface. Your body parts that are almost perpendicular to the angle of the rays receive most radiation. The shoulders and the nose burn first while you stand and, of course, most of the body is at risk while you lie on the beach. Around noon and in summer, when the sun is high in the sky, you are likely to receive the highest dose. The angle of radiation also depends on the geographical latitude. The sun's rays strike the earth's surface more directly the closer you are to the equator.
- **Ground reflection.** Most surfaces reflect only a small amount of UV radiation. The sand at the beach, however, reflects around 25% and fresh snow almost 80%. You can add these figures to the amount of radiation you receive directly from the sun.
- **Altitude.** When you are exposed to fresh snow you are probably in the mountains. With or without snow, the closer you are to the sun the higher the intensity of UV radiation. Because the earth's atmosphere rapidly thins out with altitude and the mountain air usually contains less pollution, fewer molecules are available to absorb UV radiation. For every 300 m the level increases by approximately 4%.
- **Particles in the atmosphere.** The most obvious particles are water droplets in the form of clouds—we all know how a blanket of cloud keeps a significant amount of sunlight from reaching the ground. Unfortunately, clouds don't affect UV light very much. A thin layer makes hardly any difference to the radiation level and even a thick layer can reduce it by less than 10%. Only dark storm clouds will shield you from UV radiation. If there is one good thing about pollution, it does absorb some of the UV radiation. How much is still a matter of research. On the other hand, pollution particles also scatter radiation into shady spots.
- **Water.** UV radiation penetrates the water. Almost all of it reaches to just below the surface and up to 40% penetrates to a depth of 0.5 metres.

UV radiation and human health

One important and probably only beneficial effect of UV radiation on your health is the formation of vitamin D3 in your skin. The body requires this vitamin to help with the absorption of calcium and phosphorus. If you would be without sunlight for a long time, your bones would become soft and deformed, a disease known as rickets. But as latest studies suggest, exposure of your hands and face for as little as 15 minutes per day should be sufficient to prevent the disease.

If you expose your eyes, skin and immune system to the sun, a photochemical reaction in proteins and your DNA occurs. Too much exposure to UV radiation temporarily or permanently alters the function of cell components.

In the short term, tiny blood vessels can burst and redden the skin or the eyes. Sunburn of the skin and inflammation of the eyes (e.g. snow blindness) may follow. While these effects are reversible, further exposure can lead to permanent damage, such as the clouding of eye lenses, otherwise known as cataracts. The otherwise elastic fibres of your skin thicken due to a loss of collagen and your skin ages prematurely. UV radiation can even change the genetic information stored within your DNA and may initiate cancer to the skin or the eyes. UV radiation also suppresses the immune system's ability to fight intruders such as viruses, bacteria and parasites.

'Over 2 million non-melanoma skin cancers and 200,000 malignant melanomas occur globally each year. With a 10% decrease in stratospheric ozone and current trends and behaviour, an additional 300,000 non-melanoma and 4,500 melanoma skin cancers could be expected worldwide. Some 12 to 15 million people are blind from cataracts. WHO has estimated that up to 20% of cataracts or 3 million per year could be due to UV exposure. Given that, in the United States alone, it costs the US Government $US 3.4 billion for 1.2 million cataract operations per year, substantial savings in cost to health care can be made by prevention or delay in the onset of cataracts.'

World Health Organization, 2000

Effects of UV radiation on the environment

Impact on the ecosystem

For millions of years, plants, animals and other organisms have learned to cope with UV radiation through evolutionary protection and repair. In a relatively short time, however, the human-induced depletion of the ozone layer has brought about a significant increase in UV radiation levels. The natural world has had no time to react. As a result you can hear and read some bizarre reports concerning mutated plants, blind animals and disease outbreaks.

The adverse effects of UV radiation on the ecosystem, however, develop much more subtly. Researchers have so far concentrated on individual plant or animal species and can't assess the consequences to the terrestrial or marine ecosystem as a whole. Only recently, scientists made an effort to look at the complete impact of UV radiation on the life cycle of organisms and the ecosystem. Now they seek answers on possible ill effects of UV radiation on:

- The building blocks of life such as plant cells
- Plants and animals, especially their vulnerability during immature stages
- The interactions between organisms
- The food chain and its possible implications on mankind
- Biodiversity.

Air quality

A depletion of the ozone layer allows more UV radiation to reach the lower layers of the atmosphere. In particular UVB radiation, a dominant cause of photochemical reactions, alters the chemical composition of the air.

Like the white cue ball breaks a pack of billiard balls, the energy of UVB radiation splits the bond of gas molecules. Nitrogen oxides react with volatile organic compounds and form ground level ozone (O_3), a major component of urban pollution. The ozone itself comes under attack and breaks apart, leaving three oxygen atoms (O). Their freedom is short-lived. The three rascals combine very rapidly with any available molecular oxygen (O_2), the type that we breathe, and form ozone molecules again. This process triples ozone pollution.

Other atmospheric gases, such as formaldehyde, hydrogen peroxide and nitric acid, also come under UV fire and release rogue atoms and molecules (radicals). Like the single oxygen atoms, the radicals combine with other gas molecules and increase pollution or extend the life of greenhouse gases such as methane or CFC substitutes.

Marine ecosystem

Depending on the clarity of water, UV radiation can penetrate several metres below the surface. Its damaging effect can influence organisms at depths greater than of 20 m. An increase of UV radiation starts a chain reaction within the aquatic food chain and will impact on human eating habits eventually, with less seafood being available. Some scientists claim that the chain reaction has already begun.

The first links in the food chain are phytoplankton and zooplankton. Phytoplankton are tiny plant-like organisms that float near the water surface. Like plants, they depend on the sun's light for their energy. Zooplankton, tiny animal-like organisms, hover just below phytoplankton, their source of food. The larvae of fish and crustaceans, such as shrimps, eat both organisms. They in turn have been a food source for the fish on your dinner plate.

High doses of UV radiation impacts on the phytoplankton's ability to process the sun's energy, i.e. photosynthesis. The radiation can also alter the structure of cells in plant-like and animal-like organisms and damage the eggs and larvae of fish and crustaceans. At worst, this kills a large number of them or at least has an adverse impact on growth. Thus, an increase in UV radiation will enhance the negative effect of overfishing, and regions that depend on fishing as food and employment source will suffer most.

High water temperatures are thought to be the main reason for coral bleaching. Recent experiments have found, however, that high doses of UV light also contribute to the bleaching process. Increased levels of UV radiation possibly affect the growth of algae and seagrasses as well, but this has yet to be confirmed.

Plants and animals

Stories of unexplained damage to trees, agricultural crops and other plants emerged in recent years. Researchers blame pollution, drought, diseases and the thinning of the ozone layer. Perhaps it is a combination of all. Plants are very adaptive to individual factors but how will plants cope with multiple environmental stresses?

Experimental irradiation of plants with UV shows different reactions between species. Some plants become either damaged or are limited in their growth. Others adapt or even increase their growth rate. What becomes clear, however, is that about half the tested species show some sensitivity to increased levels of UV light.

UV radiation can interfere with the plant's ability to photosynthesize by damaging or destroying chlorophyll—their green pigment—and plant cells. Stunted plants and damaged leaves are often the first signs. Like sunbathing humans, leaves, seedpods and fruit develop a suntan and get a brittle skin. Damaged leaves open the doorway to insect pests and diseases. There may also be subtle changes, such as delayed flowering and fruiting, sterility and thickening of the skin on fruit and vegetables.

As you can imagine, if one group of plants is negatively affected and the other group isn't, then the unaffected plants will eventually dominate and take over the weaklings. Is this an excuse for the weed problem on your front lawn? Not likely.

Potential UV radiation damage to plants includes:

- Disruption or prevention of the photosynthetic process
- Stunted growth
- Sterile pollen and seeds
- Adaptation processes may alter the sugar, oil and protein contents of plants
- Radiation damage to fruit and vegetables reduces quality and invites pests and diseases
- Some unwanted plant species proliferate and compete with food crops.

UV radiation has the same harmful effect on animals as it has on mankind. Frog populations are declining rapidly all over the world. Pollution, global warming and diseases are likely culprits. But a recent study points the finger at UV radiation as well. Laboratory and field studies suggest that excessive UV radiation damages the DNA in amphibian eggs.

Record levels of UV radiation may have blinded large numbers of sheep and cattle in Chile and kangaroos in Australia. Some veterinarians, however, dispute this and attribute the source to infectious diseases. Less disputed is the origin of sunburn and cataracts in some fish species that live and feed close to the water's surface.

Eye and skin diseases are also common in animals, but the number of infected animals is comparatively low. Animals are less likely to shed their protective fur, feathers or scales and sunbathe on the beach. Nevertheless, domestic stock forced to graze on fields without shaded areas have a much higher rate of skin and eye disorders than their wild cousins have.

Material damage

Since UV radiation is able to break molecules of certain atmospheric gases, it comes as no surprise that UV radiation can also degrade and destroy solid materials. Polymers, natural or synthetic chemical compounds such as rubber and all types of plastics, are particularly vulnerable. Scientists spend years to find new chemical compositions to replace expensive or heavy natural materials in household items, building materials and even aircraft and car parts. But when left in the sun long enough, they will become brittle and fall apart. Any increase in UV radiation will shorten the life of these materials further. To extend the life of products, manufacturers need to add expensive stabilizing chemicals.

SKIN DISORDERS

UV radiation and the skin

Your skin is like a shopping bag full of goodies. Both prevent their valuable contents from spilling on to the ground. But the skin also

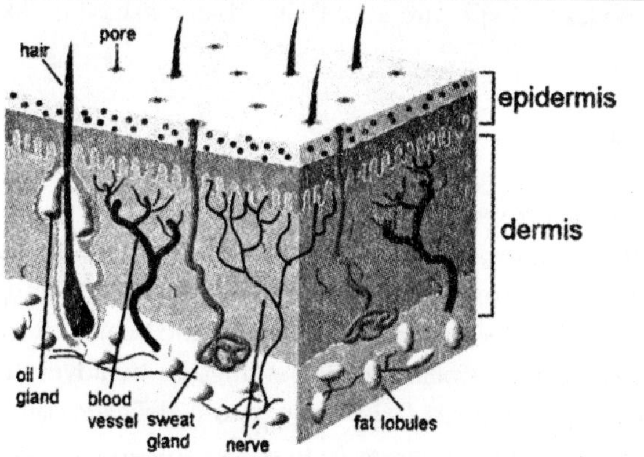

protects you against the intrusion of harmful substances, organisms and radiation.

The outer layer, epidermis, takes most punishment. It is insensitive and contains no blood vessels. Unfortunately it is also very thin, so pain and damage easily reach the lower layer—the dermis. Nerve fibre, blood vessels, hair roots, sweat glands, DNA and collagen fibres, to name a few, are located in this layer. If your skin is unprotected, UV radiation penetrates deep into the dermis.

Your skin is able to defend against mild radiation attacks. Skin cells produce melanin, the substance that tans your skin. Suntan is a weak shield against the harmful radiation—some skin cells die during the battle and form a protective horny layer of dead tissue. The skin repairs most damage to the cells and discards the victims. In your lifetime you shed approximately 18kg of skin.

Frequent exposure or high doses of UV radiation may lead to temporary or permanent changes to your skin, passing sunburn being a painful indicator. Too much damage will show up in wrinkles and dry skin. These are the signs of damage to the collagen fibres. The skin ages prematurely and permanently—photoageing. A billion-dollar cosmetic industry tries to sell products that promise to prevent, minimize or repair the damage, or at least hide it.

DNA is the 'repair manual' of the skin. UV radiation is capable of seriously distorting the information contained in the DNA instruction book, however, and the repair process may not proceed on its intended path and could instead lead to skin cancer. Skin cancer occurs mostly in fair-skinned people, but it is uncertain whether prolonged exposure, high doses or exposure at childhood increases the risk.

Suntan

'Look how brown you are. You must have had a good holiday.' Fair-skinned people are still obsessed with the need to have a suntanned skin on return from their annual holidays. Their friends and colleagues regard a tanned skin as a sign of health and beauty. A man with a tawny, weather-beaten appearance is assumed to be adventurous and strong, while a pale-skinned fellow suggests a delicate constitution. While it may be quite an adventure to find a vacant spot on the beach between thousands of fellow sunbathers, the bronzed hero is unlikely to have ever ventured from the coast.

The trend is to have a tan all year round. Tanning devices and creams become increasingly popular, and while creams are safe, tanning beds aren't. Manufacturers try to explain that their product transmits mainly 'good' UVA light. Scientists, however, do not find any 'goodness' in UVA radiation. It penetrates the skin even deeper than UVB light and is said to negatively influence the body's immune system.

Tanning occurs in two steps: immediate pigment darkening and delayed tanning. The skin cells always contain some melanin that darkens within 5 to 10 minutes after exposure to UV radiation but may fade within less than 2 hours. UV radiation also triggers the production of more melanin and it darkens deeper layers of the skin. Delayed tanning continues over the next 2–3 days and the result persists for many weeks.

A tanned skin and the development of dead tissue on its surface are a defence mechanism against excessive UV radiation. UV radiation protection from a tan is only moderate, though. A much better protection—and much less attractive—results in the thickening of the outer layer of the skin.

Sunburn

The Australian Defence Force issues soldiers with the means to protect themselves from harmful UV radiation, making severe sunburn a form of negligence and self-inflicted injury that requires a reprimand. It seems a fair argument: by now, everyone should be aware of UV radiation dangers and should either pay attention to the body's warning signals or at least learn from the first painful experience.

Tiny blood vessels in an unprotected skin become damaged and burst. In less than 4 hours, the radiated area becomes red and tender. If the affected person would 'listen' to his or her body and move into the shade, the effect would fade within 1–2 days. But if the person refuses to take notice, UV radiation penetrates deep into the skin where it destroys many cells. The skin desperately tries to prevent damage by thickening the outer layer and reacts violently with painful fluid-filled blisters. After a few days of healing, the dead skin peels off. Frequent sunburns will continuously shorten the time between exposure and the appearance of the first symptoms.

The severity and onset of sunburn depends, amongst other factors, on the skin type. Many fair-skinned people experience a reaction to UV radiation within less than half an hour, whereas people with a dark skin may not sunburn at all.

Photoageing

Loose, dry, rough and leathery skin; deep wrinkles and furrows; skin that is unevenly pigmented and covered in brown freckles or other blemishes; if that's what your skin will look like at old age, you have done well. Many others reach this weather-beaten look at the age of 30 or 40. Photoaged skin is the term for the signs and symptoms and photoageing describes the process.

Too much sunshine changes the structure of the skin permanently and is responsible for premature skin blemishes such as:

- **Wrinkles.** UV radiation damages collagen fibres. The repair process becomes rather disorganized and collagen fibres form where they shouldn't, resulting in wrinkles.
- **Solar elastosis.** Damage to collagen triggers additional production of elastin. Excess elastin stretches the skin and forces it to sag and form furrows. The skin of the neck and the upper back are usually the least protected and suffer most.
- **Stellate** or **sun scars.** Excessive exposure to the sun takes its toll on sweat and oil glands. They are no longer able to function efficiently, thus depriving the skin of moisture. The skin becomes dry, thick, scaly and scars easily. Wounds tend to heal slowly.
- **Solar** or **senile purpura.** The fine blood vessels in overexposed skin rupture quite easily, resulting in slow-healing bruises, especially on the hands and forearms. The bruises can look alarming but are generally harmless.
- **Freckles** (also named **liver** or **age spots**) can occur at any age. They are most common on the fair skin of children and of adults over the age of 55, particularly on the sun-exposed skin such as hands, face, arms and shoulders. These flat brown or black spots can be tiny or

several centimetres in diameter. Cosmetics can either hide the blemishes or bleach the colour.

- **Solar comedones.** A little more annoying than freckles are solar comedones, pimples that look like acne but are not related. The blemish is also known as Favre-Racouchet disease. The pimples occur predominately on the face and are either open (blackheads) or closed (whiteheads). Comedones develop after considerable exposure to UV radiation and appear more often on the skin of heavy smokers.

Of course, this process doesn't happen overnight. The effects accumulate over the years and the result depends very much on the frequency and intensity of exposure to UV radiation. While heat, wind, and air pollutants also accelerate photoageing, UV radiation is to blame for about 90% of the symptoms.

People with a fair complexion living in sun-drenched countries are at highest risk of developing photoaged skin. Included in the high-risk group are farmers, fishermen, outdoor workers and sunbathers. In other words, everyone is at risk who spends much time in the sun. Heavy smoking and pollution appear to make matters worse.

Less UV radiation will delay photoageing. But try telling your son or daughter to take it easy on the obligatory suntan. Most aren't interested in what happens at the 'old' age of 30 or 40 and assume that if all fails, 'they' will come up with something. 'They' are the cosmetic industries and medical specialists (dermatologists). Indeed, there are many diets, drugs, ointments, treatments and surgical methods—some may actually work.

Cosmetic companies battle for the right to claim a cure for photoageing. Some swear on the application of products containing vitamins such as A, C, or E. Others convince customers that antioxidants and oestrogen are the solution. Another way of reducing wrinkles is to shed some of the dead tissue on the skin's surface. You can accomplish this by applying over-the-counter scrubs and peels lotions that contain acids such as alpha hydroxyl acid. Your skin specialist can apply stronger acids for a better result but chemical peeling isn't without side effects.

Specialists can also fill the trenches in your face with animal collagen or with your own body fat, or they can grind down the ridges with abrasive tools or lasers. A third technique, cosmetic surgery, requires incisions and can correct larger furrows or folds. Sounds like work on a construction site?

Photosensitivity

It is spring at last: you get out your shorts or swimsuit and are determined to enjoy the first warm and sunny days. Curiously, after just a short while and despite sunscreen, your skin starts to itch and turns red in patches. Some tiny blisters or pimples also spring up. No wonder, you kept your skin covered for a long time over winter and your skin has become light sensitive. In this scenario, the symptoms are probably only temporary and will disappear once your skin gets used to the UV radiation.

Others are not so fortunate. Even low levels of light, as during wintertime, can trigger minor or major reactions. These people suffer from photosensitivity. As with allergies, a variety of substances or disorders can trigger the symptoms. It can be something such as food or medication, or it can be a skin-care product. Certain medical conditions trigger photosensitivity or UV radiation can aggravate the condition.

The number of cases with mild to moderate photosensitivity is not easily established. Minor symptoms are often mistaken for a typical reaction to UV radiation, such as sunburn. This can be very tricky when a sunburnt person tries to counter the effects by applying a sunscreen that may contain sensitivity-increasing chemicals.

Substances causing photosensitivity

- **Medication** taken internally or applied externally can cause photosensitivity. This includes drugs such as high blood pressure treatments, antiseptic creams, birth control pills, antihistamines, antibiotics, pain relievers, diuretics, antidepressants, antidiabetics, anti-inflammatory and cancer treatment drugs.
- Some **herbal remedies** and essential oils can have the same effect. St. John's wort and bergamot essential oil have been known to cause photosensitivity in humans and animals.
- **Food.** Some people eat a stick of celery and develop a 'sunburn.'

Hard to swallow, but it's true. Many types of food can trigger photosensitivity but the most common culprits are parsley, carrots, celery, mustard, limes and figs.

- **Skin care products.** Chemicals in substances that get into contact with the skin can cause photosensitivity and a variety of symptoms. Often they are 'hidden' in products such as soaps, perfumes, shampoos, skin lotions, aftershaves, detergents and even sunscreen containing para-aminobenzonic acid or certain fragrances.

Medical conditions causing photosensitivity

- **Porphyria** is a metabolic disorder causing an overproduction of porphyrins (chemical compounds). The blood carries some of the excess porphyrin to the skin where it accumulates and causes extreme photosensitivity. Symptoms range from redness and blisters to permanent scarring.
- **Lupus** (lupus erythematosus) is a disease where the immune system becomes confused and attacks the body's own tissue instead of intruding organisms. The disease affects women more often than it does men. Amongst other problems, the skin becomes sensitive to UV radiation, causing skin rashes and fever.
- **Xeroderma pigmentosa.** A beautiful sunny day invites everyone to outdoor activities. For sufferers of xeroderma pigmentosa, however, every ray of sunshine increases the chance of skin cancer by a thousand times. Even the light that penetrates the windows is enough to bring about sunburn or blistering. Patients are normally confined indoors and if they venture outside they either have to wear a protective suit or apply sunscreen with the highest possible protection factor. People with xeroderma pigmentosa inherit an inability to repair UV radiation damage to their DNA. Fortunately the incidence of this disease is less than 2 per 100,000 people.

Disorders resulting from photosensitivity

- **Polymorphis light eruption** is a fancy name for rashes. It is the most common disorder associated with photosensitivity and affects an estimated 10% of US citizens and around 20% of Swedes. The real number is probably higher as most minor occurrences aren't reported.

The disorder appears in all races, but more frequently in fair-skinned women.

Burning or itching rashes, consisting of red spots, patches or blisters, show within 1 to 4 days of exposure to UV radiation, usually on arms and lower legs. If the person avoids further exposure, the symptoms disappear within a couple of weeks but can recur after another exposure. But because the skin adapts to sunlight, the effects should become less severe every time.

- **Chronic photosensitivity dermatitis**, also known as chronic actinic dermatitis, is another result of photosensitivity. It is widespread, but this time affects elderly male more often than it does women. Inflamed and itchy patches appear on the exposed skin. Scales and pimples can accompany the eczema.
- **Sun hives (solar urticaria)** is a rare skin condition. It usually doesn't comprise more than 5% of all photosensitive skin disorders. People of all races, age and gender can contract this disease. Its symptoms are usually red swollen patches that intensely sting or itch.

Non-cancerous growths

Moles

The dictionary offers several meanings for a mole. Amidst others, it can be a deceiving infiltrator, someone who hides amongst a group of people to secretly further the interests of a rival party. So does the skin cancer melanoma. It lurks behind the mask of one of many harmless skin blemishes.

The majority of skin moles, however, are benign skin-coloured or brown to black bumps. They are there since birth or appear later in life, especially after extensive exposure to UV radiation. Moles are rare amongst dark-skinned people but are very common on fair skins.

Watch that mole

Be suspicious if the mole:

- changes colour
- is of different colour to others
- increases in size
- has an irregular outline
- has crusts
- bleeds or oozes
- itches or is painful.

People with many moles are at a higher risk of developing skin cancer than are people with low numbers of moles. In addition, moles are easily mistaken for melanoma. Medical practitioners are, therefore, becoming increasingly cautious. They either closely monitor changes in appearance or cut a sample for a microscopic analysis. They sometimes completely remove a mole if it develops into a cancer suspect or into a nuisance.

Venous Lake

UV radiation damages the tiny blood vessels in the skin. In this case it is the veins that dilate and form small dark-blue or violet 'lakes.' Venous lakes appear as soft and compressible bumps on the sun-exposed skin of the face, neck and ears. Although common, it develops more often in the elderly. Race appears to be no factor. Some medical scientists support the theory that blood clotting (thrombosis) is at least partially to blame.

Like moles, other than being a cosmetic nuisance, venous lakes are harmless and painless. On the other hand venous lake can look similar to skin cancer. A microscopic analysis prevents a misdiagnosis.

Solar keratosis

Solar keratosis is also known as actinic keratosis. It is not a skin cancer but is a common pre-cancerous condition caused by excessive UV radiation. Early diagnosis and treatment is important. Minor surgery with scalpel, laser or chemicals can remove the growth.

Horny, scaly bumps on sun-exposed skin are the first signs. They can become tender and quite aggressive. At this stage, solar keratosis has an estimated 10% chance of evolving into cancer. Because the damaging effect of UV radiation adds up over a lifetime, the elderly—particularly if they are fair-skinned—are the most likely victims. Due to the modern suntan culture, however, the number of patients of a younger age has increased steadily, with people in their early twenties now being diagnosed with some form of solar keratosis.

Keratoacanthoma

If solar keratosis doesn't fool your medical practitioner into diagnosing you with skin cancer, then keratoacanthoma might. This skin blemish can look exactly like non-melanoma skin cancer and is clinically not different to one of its manifestations. Keratoacanthoma begins its life as a small pimple but, if untreated, grows very rapidly into an unsightly crater, often with a solid crusty core.

Again, UV radiation plays a major role. A minor injury, however, appears to trigger the growth. Keratoacanthoma's big difference to real cancer is that is self-healing: once it reaches its maximum growth it begins a cycle of self-destruction and disappears within a few months. The growth is often surgically removed before it leaves an ugly scar. Keratoacanthoma is less common in dark-skinned people.

Skin cancer

Today skin cancer is more prevalent than all other human cancers combined. Is the weather to blame? Yes and no. UV radiation is undoubtedly a major trigger of skin cancer. But equal blame goes to a change in contemporary human behaviour, as more leisure time and the desire for a tan lead to more radiation exposure.

Despite education and early detection programmes, numbers of skin cancer patients are rapidly increasing everywhere. Fortunately, an average of about 95% of diagnoses is of the less lethal non-melanoma type. The sun-soaked Australians hold the infamous world record for the highest melanoma rate, at 9.6% of total national cancer cases against just 2.1% in Europe. Numbers of melanoma cases in the US are halfway between the Australian and European rates.

Two types of non-melanoma skin cancer are common: basal cell carcinoma (BCC) and squamous cell carcinoma (SCC). Both are seldom a threat to life. If removed at an early stage and with good medical care, the mortality rate is less than 1%. Nevertheless, they can severely damage the skin. Because both occur mostly on the visible sun-exposed body parts, in particular the head and neck, the cancers can disfigure a person's appearance.

BCC is the least aggressive of the two. It rarely spreads to other body sites. Though almost always curable, the cancer is recurring. SCC is slightly more aggressive and has the potential to spread. BCC often appears as shiny, waxy red bumps. SCC shows itself more likely as red and scaly bumps. But both cancers can take many forms. At times, they become non-healing open sores.

Less common but more dangerous is melanoma. It usually develops on sun-exposed body parts but can appear in different forms anywhere on the body, even in the eye. Unfortunately, it very often looks like a benign mole somewhere on the skin (see 'Non-cancerous growth' p. 122). The cancer readily spreads via lymph and blood vessels to other body tissue or organs. In almost a quarter of melanoma cases, the survival rate is low.

Both cancer types, non-melanoma and melanoma, can arise from sun damage. You read earlier that UV radiation scrambles the chemical code of skin cells—the DNA. The skin's repair system can no longer read the code and generates an out-of-control malignant growth. In some cases, UV radiation is only the trigger and the repair system could have inherited a genetic fault that prevents it from properly reading the code. Other possible causes are a suppressed or defective immune system and certain toxic substances.

Fair-skinned and light-haired people lack the amount of skin pigments, melanin, that provide a protective shield against UV radiation. Skin cancer is, therefore, much more prominent in such populations, although not exclusively. Other genetic factors that are related to an increased risk are a tendency to sunburn instead of tanning, and a high number of moles.

Accumulated UV radiation is the main cause of non-melanoma type skin cancer in the elderly. A lifetime of excessive sun exposure, however, does not explain why melanoma grows very often on unexposed skin areas, such as the legs and the trunk. One theory is that short, frequent and intense exposure of non-acclimatized skin, especially at childhood, is likely to blame. Playing or sunbathing at the beach are examples. The figures from Australia show that the risk further increases if a person lives and works in a sunny country.

Treatment depends on the stage of the cancer and the health of the patient. In the early stages, surgery best prevents further growth but advanced skin cancer requires additional treatment, the most common being chemotherapy, despite its unwelcome side effects. Unfortunately, chemotherapy is not a cure. It can at best shrink the cancer or at worst slow the growth for a few months. Radiating the cancer is another common therapy. The procedure also tries to shrink or destroy the growth. Non-melanoma type skin cancer often responds quite well, but melanoma cells are more resistant.

Since the body has its own defences against cancerous growth, it seems logical that doctors work on a way to support a patient's immune system. First trials show that once a person responds to an experimental drug treatment, the benefits last much longer than they do with chemotherapy. Several natural products, such as herbal supplements, also aim to support the immune system, but their long-term benefits are so far unknown. Gene therapy has a similar purpose: like reloading a corrupt computer program, the right genes replace the faulty inherited material.

Skin cancer research is of national importance to many countries. Government agencies and industry both frantically search for cancer cures. Regardless of whether the motive is to save money in national health programmes or to make money by selling the cancer-curing 'wonder drug', we all will benefit eventually. In the meantime, the public can either blame the weather or follow the many preventative measures as published by health agencies.

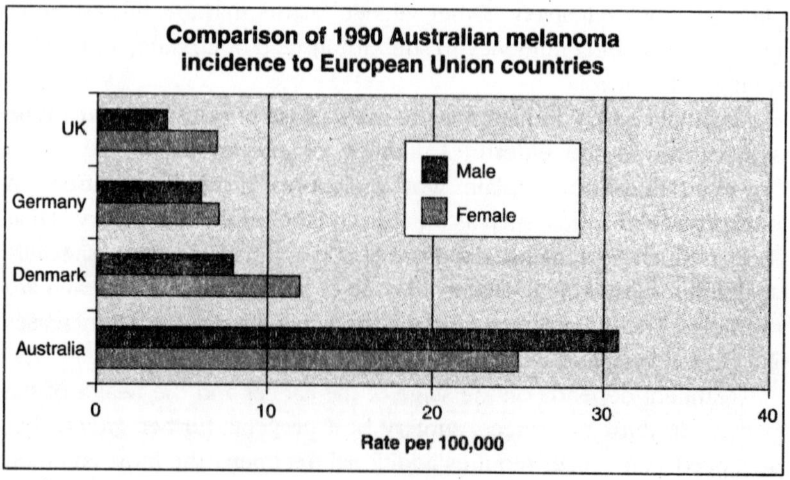

EYE DISORDERS

Sunlight and the eye

Take a table-tennis ball and name its skin sclera; line the interior with a light-sensitive film and name it retina; cut a hole and name it pupil; insert a lens and name it lens; place a circular shutter in front of the lens and name it iris; protect the lens and shutter with some clear plastic and name it cornea. There you are: you have created a model of a very primitive eye.

Instead of a layer of light-sensitive material, the human retina contains many light-sensing nerves. They translate the different wavelengths of visible light into coded signals. Most nerves are at and near the centre of your eyes' back walls, the areas for sharp vision. Eye professionals call it macula. The optic nerve transmits the coded signals to your brain. Since birth, the brain learned to interpret the signals and form images in your mind.

Like so many other body parts, the eyes wear out with age and you can expedite the ageing process by allowing UV radiation damage. You will only notice the damage when it is too late though, when your vision is no longer good. And if you are very careless, you don't have to wait that long: gazing at the sun can cause immediate damage.

The tissue at the front of your eyes absorbs most of the UV radiation, but at a cost. The tissue cells may alter their structure or become damaged, just like the skin cells do. While the skin has its tanning and dead skin cell layer as defences against radiation, the eyes don't have this protection. They only rely on your eyelids to close when the light is too bright. Unfortunately, because you can't see UV light, the reflex of closing your eyelids only works in combination with bright visible light.

Despite just a small percentage of UV light reaching the interior of your eye, it is still enough to slowly destroy some of the light-sensitive nerves on the retina. This is particularly true for the macula, the area of sharp vision (see 'Macular Degeneration' p. 128). So, whenever you can, keep the harmful rays out by wearing UV-blocking sunglasses.

UV radiation damage can show itself in many forms:

- **Degeneration.** UV radiation accelerates the ageing process. Macular degeneration, the damage to the central part of the retina, is a leading cause of blindness in many countries. Degeneration of the cornea, droplet keratopathy, is common in populations in areas of high UV exposure.

- **Sunburn.** Sunlight can burn your eye as well as your skin. The cornea becomes inflamed and very painful (photokeratitis). While corneal injury is only temporary, a burn to the retina is permanent and affects the vision.
- **Cataracts.** Overexposure to UV light can cause clouding of the lens.
- **Non-cancerous growth.** UV radiation is said to trigger pterygium and pinguecula, fleshy growths in the corner of the eye. Normally both are harmless, but pterygium can invade the cornea and cause vision impairment.
- **Cancer.** Though rare, all types of skin cancer can affect the eye.

UV radiation damage to the eyes does not distinguish between races. The number of incidents is directly related to sun exposure. Recreational activities in snow, at the beach and on or near water, without adequate protection, increase the risk. Living and working in countries with high doses of UV radiation sees the numbers rise further.

Degeneration

The toddler squeals happily in its pram when it sees the images of butterflies and birds in a blue sky. Of course, it can't see the UV radiation coming the other way. Mum should know better. But have you seen proper sunglasses for infants? Overexposure at early childhood lays the foundation for prematurely aged eyes. Nevertheless, while the eyes are particularly vulnerable during childhood development, UV radiation damage occurs at any age and it accumulates.

Macular Degeneration

You need the macula, the central vision, to read, write, drive and watch television. In other words, the macula provides you with the ability to see fine details. Macular degeneration is an irreversible damage to the light-sensing nerves. Don't confuse this with farsightedness, which affects the lens and is easily corrected with reading glasses.

Age is the main risk factor in macular degeneration. One estimate puts the number of affected US citizens at approximately 10% of people in the 52 to 65 age group. Around half of the population over 75 has some form of macular degeneration. This number will rise with the overall increase in life expectancy.

Several other factors contribute to macular degeneration. The case against UV radiation, and most recently against blue and violet light, is continually strengthening. Bright light straight from the sun, or from reflective surfaces such as the ocean, snow or sand will 'age' the macula. It also doesn't help to be a male smoker with a fair complexion, to be on certain medications, or to have parents and grandparents with macular degeneration.

The patient doesn't lose vision completely, as the disorder doesn't generally affect the peripheral and colour vision. But he or she will have a distorted or blank area in the centre of their vision, just like looking through spectacles with water droplets on their lenses' centre. The droplets are clear at first but steadily become murky. This common 'dry' type of macular degeneration generally progresses slowly. An eye specialist often discovers these deposits before they affect the vision. Much more serious and rapid is the 'wet' type of macular degeneration. Here, leaking and bleeding blood vessels grow underneath the macula, lifting it up and causing nerve cells to die.

The loss of vision can't be repaired but certain precautions, such as UV radiation protection, improved fitness and a healthy lifestyle and diet can slow the progress. A surgical technique called laser photocoagulation may be able to destroy or block some of the leaking blood vessels before they become harmful. A new drug therapy aims for the same target. Also, some optical devices may help to shift the centre of vision to unaffected areas.

Droplet Keratopathy

The case against UV radiation is much stronger in relation to droplet keratopathy. An alternative name, climatic droplet keratopathy, clearly makes such a suggestion. This condition is a major cause of blindness in populations of arctic regions and tropical islands—in circumstances where reflections from snow, sand and water intensify the sunlight. Of course, overexposure increases the risk regardless of geographical location.

UV radiation alters proteins in the cornea. The protein takes on the form of translucent and sometimes yellowish droplets. They make the light rays refract, resulting in blurred vision. Surgeons are able to remove some of the droplets.

Sunburn

Solar Maculopathy

The lens of your eye is no different to a magnifying glass that bundles the sun's rays and sets a piece of paper alight. In the case of the eye, only around 20 seconds of sun gazing is enough to burn the back of your eyeball, the macula. The time is even shorter if you are foolish enough to look at the sun with binoculars or a telescope.

Millions of people, however, are so foolhardy during solar eclipses when they stare at the phenomenon without proper eye protection—and many get hurt. Even the rays of a partially eclipsed sun are strong enough to inflict permanent damage. This happens so often that a common name for the injury is eclipse burn. Eclipses aren't the only opportunities for those seconds of folly. People with temporary mental disorders, as during drug and alcohol abuse, or with psychiatric problems, may lose the common sense to avoid sun gazing.

In extreme cases, the bundled light permanently destroys the delicate light-sensing layer on the retina and leaves a blind area. In milder cases, the beam impairs the ability to sense light, but its function restores after a short time.

Solar maculopathy is sometimes called solar retinopathy because it often affects the peripheral vision as well. It doesn't warn you of the damage, as the retina has no pain-sensing nerves. But after a short while the following untreatable symptoms may appear:

- Temporary or permanent loss of central or peripheral vision
- Distorted or blurred vision
- Dark patches in the field of vision
- Unusual colours
- Light sensitivity
- Sore eyes.

Photokeratitis

Photokeratitis is the medical term for a sunburnt eye and snow blindness. The front of your eyeball, the cornea, is subjected to high levels of UV radiation in mountain areas, on snowfields and on sandy beaches. Around two hours on snow and six hours on sand are enough to burn the eyes.

Unlike solar maculopathy, sunburnt eyes hurt. The pain can be severe but usually doesn't occur until several hours later and a 'snow-blind' skier may blame the late night instead. Even the additional symptoms of red eyes, swollen eyelids, light sensitivity and blurred vision may not convince the person of the real cause. In any case, photokeratitis is not permanent. The affected eyes should fully recover within a few days.

Light sensitivity

Does bright light bother you? If so, it doesn't necessarily indicate a problem. Many people weep in bright sunlight, especially if reflective surfaces are present. If you visit an eye specialist, you probably experience light sensitivity afterwards if they have used some eye drops to dilate your pupils for the examination. As a result, more light can penetrate deep into your eyes, which is uncomfortable, sometimes painful, and may bring out some tears. Bright light is a trigger of migraine and headache in some people.

Light sensitivity, also called photophobia, is a common disorder and in some cases is the symptom of another problem. The light-sensitive person may have a medical disorder that triggers light sensitivity, or he or she reacts to certain drugs or toxins.

Cataracts

When your fingerprints are all over the lens of your camera, the pictures you take won't be as sharp as expected. You won't let this happen to your eyes, I guess. Nevertheless, the lens of your eye can become hazy for other reasons. One of them is the fine weather.

Ageing is the main reason for the clouding of the lens, but excessive UV radiation of a clear

Cataract symptoms

- Blurred or hazy vision
- Poor night vision
- Glare from very bright light
- Halos around lights
- Light sensitivity
- Dull colours
- Double vision
- Improved close vision (temporary)

blue sky is another major contributor. The World Health Organization estimates that cataracts account for almost 15 million blind people worldwide. About 20%, or 3 million, of these are most likely caused by UV radiation.

> **Cataracts are caused by:**
>
> - Age
> - UV radiation
> - Heredity
> - Eye injury or inflammation
> - Toxins
> - Diabetes
> - Alcohol and nicotine abuse
> - Excessive heat
> - Certain drugs and medication.

The lens is not solid. It is a capsule filled with water and protein fibres. The protein fibres are normally crystal clear but can 'wear out' with age. They can become opaque, similar to how an egg white clouds when it gets cooked. Other factors, such as UV radiation, can alter the protein prematurely.

Cataract development is very variable amongst individuals. The process is generally slow and initially may affect only part of the lens. In one person it develops from the lens's rim and grows inside, in another person's eye the lens begins to cloud from the centre. Curiously, when the centre is lightly clouded, the person may temporarily improve the ability to see close objects. In any case, the growing cataract will eventually severely impair vision and frequently lead to blindness.

In the early stages, a cataract is merely a nuisance. But soon extra lighting, different eyeglasses and protection from glare is needed. UV radiation protection and less alcohol and nicotine should help to slow the process. Some swear on the effectiveness of alternative supplements and diets.

Once the cataract interferes too much with the daily life, surgery should be considered. Eye surgeons replace millions of cloudy lenses with substitutes every year, and this safe procedure returns better vision to as much as 90% of patients.

Non-cancerous growth

Sunlight helps to grow many useful things in nature but sun also has to take the blame for some rather useless growth on your eyeballs. When someone tries to convince you again that everything in life has its purpose, point to either corner of your eye and ask the smart person, 'What purpose does this fatty, fleshy growth have, then?'

Pterygium and pingueculum are the names for common but harmless yellow-white growths. Both are almost identical in appearance and usually begin their lives on the nasal side of the eyes. They slowly grow towards the centre, but only pterygium may encroach onto the cornea and cause vision problems.

Because UV radiation is a major factor, the disorder occurs mostly in populations of 'sun-drenched' countries. Heat, wind and airborne irritants can inflame the growth. Anti-inflammatory eye drops reduce the redness and itching. Otherwise, treatment is not necessary unless the growth affects vision or is cosmetically undesirable.

Eye cancer

The eyes aren't immune against cancer. Squamous and basal cell cancer often develop on the sun-exposed parts such as the cornea and the eyelids. As previously mentioned, body parts perpendicular to the sun's rays are most at risk of UV radiation damage, so therefore the lower eyelid margin suffers most. Symptoms and treatment are similar to skin cancer.

A malignant melanoma can start its destructive life on about every part of the eye. It can even hide behind the skin of the retina. Sunlight is again a prominent risk factor, especially overexposure to it in early life. It comes as no surprise that populations in countries with high UV radiation levels have most victims.

IMMUNE SYSTEM

UV Radiation and the immune system

Do you get apprehensive when someone with a needle comes too close? Not many people want their skin poked with sharp instruments. But what about the things you don't see: bacteria, viruses, fungi and parasites. If these organisms were of a visible size, you and I would go crazy. Millions of these aliens try to invade our body every day. Lucky for us, our creator thought of something to keep the intruders at bay—the immune system.

A healthy immune system grows the right amount of 'killer' cells that chomp away on anything foreign to your body. Outside influences or genetic disorders, however, can either damage the immune system or instruct it to ignore intruders. A person with such a defect is at risk of developing severe diseases more often and with greater severity than a healthy person does. A faulty immune system also loses the ability to control cancer. Even more disturbing are the latest findings that a suppressed immune system may diminish the desired effect of vaccination programmes.

The body has two immune systems:

- **Humoral immunity** acts by creating antibodies within a person's body fluids such as the blood
- **Cellular immunity** is based on the action of specific cells that eliminate intruders.

The second system relies on a large number of 'police' cells (Langerhans cells) in the skin to detect foreign substances. Once detected, they inform the thymus gland to release 'executioner' cells (T-cells). They don't bring an axe or a rope; instead they use the help of a form of white blood cells (macrophages)—the 'killer' cells. They engulf and digest the intruders. The macrophages present the leftovers to 'memory' T-cells, which keep records of the invaders. The next time the same type of invader shows up, the immune system responds much faster and more efficiently. Does this sound like a science-fiction thriller?

This system works quite well—most of the time. UV radiation, however, is capable of destroying many of the Langerhans cells, so intruders can invade undetected. The thymus gland may even become so confused by strong sunlight that it sends out 'messenger' T-cells to stop the 'executioner' cells from doing their work (photoimmunosuppression). As a result, the cellular immune system becomes tolerant to certain organisms. This time, the fair-skinned person is not the only type at risk. All skin types respond similarly.

A vaccination introduces a certain virus or bacteria to your immune system, such as an influenza or measles virus. Sounds scary, but this intruder is either dead or very weak and can't do much harm. The immune system destroys the intruder and stores the relevant information for later use. You are now immune against this particular strand of virus—so you hope.

Unfortunately, your habit of sunbathing just prior to the vaccination may have suppressed your immune system enough to make the procedure useless. That sounds farfetched, but recent experimental models confirm the theory. The World Health Organization warns that vaccination programmes in populations with high UV radiation exposure can be ineffective. Furthermore, some animal studies found that instead of becoming immune, the recipient of the vaccine becomes tolerant and more susceptible to the disease.

Infectious diseases

Animal experiments in laboratories show that UV radiation suppresses the immune system. Research is under way to confirm the belief of many immunologists that humans are affected in the same manner. Because UV radiation is believed to affect only the cells in sun-exposed body parts—skin and eyes—the cellular immune system is the likely victim of radiation damage. Consequently, organisms gain easy access to your body via the skin.

Measles, chicken pox, herpes and HIV viruses find it easier to proliferate in radiation-damaged cells. Animal and preliminary human studies found that even latent viruses can be activated by UV radiation. To prove the point, researchers exposed patients with previous cold sores on the lips to UV radiation. At first, they were given a sunscreen to cover the lips. None developed the symptoms of cold sores. After the same test, but with a fake sunscreen, around three-quarters of patients developed cold sores—the virus became active again. Tests with mice, meanwhile, showed a reactivation of HIV viruses after UV radiation exposure. A radiation-damaged immune system is also to blame for slower than normal clearances of parasitic infections of rodents, such as malaria, leishmaniasis, and trichinosis.

Like it or not, bacteria and fungi have a permanent place on and in your skin. A suppressed immune system allows the organisms to proliferate, however, and become a major health problem.

CIRCADIAN RHYTHM DISORDERS

Daily and seasonal changes in light intensity drive most of your automatic and hormonal body functions. They influence the 'internal clock'—the circadian rhythm. One obvious response of this 'clock' to light changes is to regulate the sleep-wake cycle. But amongst other functions, it also controls the rhythmic fluctuations in body temperature, mood and behaviour.

The production of the hormone melatonin in the pineal gland, a small and specialized organ in the brain, varies with daylight hours. The gland is most active at night and least active at day. The hormone informs other body parts of the length of daylight and darkness periods and of the light intensity. The body reacts appropriately to the environmental circumstances with, for example, tiredness or a change in body temperature.

In October 2000, the *New England Journal of Medicine* published a study in which scientists tested melatonin supplements on a small group of blind people. This group of people suffered from sleep disorders because they could not distinguish between light and dark. After taking the supplement, the majority of the participants developed normal sleep cycles.

But you don't have to be blind to disrupt your biological clock. Air travel and irregular shift work confuse the sleep-wake cycle resulting in either jet lag or sleep problems. Treatment with melatonin supplements may help.

Seasonal Affective Disorder (SAD)

Grey and rainy days make a mockery of UV radiation-related skin and eye disorders. 'Skin cancer because of sunlight? I don't even know what the sun looks like,' you joke. The sun-related dangers to your health are less, but instead your mood declines with every grey day. You are lethargic and you long for hibernation rather than work. You are a victim of the 'winter blues'.

Light plays an important role in the biological rhythm of humans. For you, this syndrome may be nothing else than the cause for a bad mood and hopefully doesn't affect your daily life. But up to 5% of people living in areas with seasonal low light suffer from the more serious seasonal affective disorder (SAD).

Well, here is something you really want to blame on the weather. Oversleeping, lethargy, weight gain, craving for sweets are some of the mild symptoms of SAD or the 'winter blues'. For some, however, the disorder can also show itself in severe depression. The very unfortunate are no longer able to work effectively and lose all interest in social activities.

The disorder affects women more often than it does men: about three-quarters of all patients are women of all age groups. Less daylight during winter appears to be the major trigger of SAD, rather than short-term dull weather. Some very sensitive persons experience the symptoms also in spring and summer during cloudy days and even inside poorly lit buildings.

Variations in light intensity alter hormone levels. In the evening the level of melatonin increases, but drops off again in the morning. During the day, the level of serotonin hormones is at its peak. But which hormone is ultimately to blame for depressive mood changes is still unclear.

If a lack of light can create such problems then bright light should prevent it. Many cultures from latitudes with long winters must know this. They light bonfires to drive away the 'evil spirits', or go on vacations to sunnier places. A little more sophisticated and effective are modern light therapies. Many patients respond well to short periods of high-intensity light exposure. In most cases the next spring or summer brings back the energy and a happy mood.

BE SUN-SMART

To a certain extent, your skin can slowly adapt to UV radiation. A horny layer and darkening gives you some protection against the harmful rays—but not enough. Overexposure can still lead to many skin, eye and immune system disorders. Prevention is much easier, cheaper and less painful than treatment.

You shouldn't lock yourself in a dark room, though. Measured exposure to sunshine is necessary to sustain life—your life. But what is too much sunshine?

There is no easy answer. Every person reacts differently to UV radiation. With an equal amount of radiation, some develop sunburn within minutes while others take hours. Always err on the safe side, especially if you are in a high-risk group. A respect for UV radiation is the key to sun-smart behaviour.

Health authorities should:

- Create an awareness in the public, especially children, of the adverse effects of UV radiation and encourage sun-smart behaviour
- Establish education programmes for employers, teachers, health care professionals, etc
- Support the use of a universal solar index by the media. The following is an internationally accepted index indicating exposure levels:

0–2	minimal
3–4	low
5–6	moderate
7–9	high
10+	very high

- Share research and statistics with other countries
- Provide sun shelters in public areas
- Establish standards for sun protection measures, such as sunscreens and sunglasses
- Finance research to establish a better understanding of the mechanisms in sun-induced disorders, particularly skin cancer, cataracts and damages to the immune system.

Behaviour

Many governments educate their citizens comprehensively about the dangers of excessive UV radiation. Most Australians, for instance, are well aware of the dangers. But the belief that a suntan is healthy and attractive is still deeply engraved in the minds of the population. Women are generally more likely to obtain a suntan as a fashion statement. For many men, a suntan and leathery skin still represents the image of a rugged and healthy outdoor type. Youngsters spend more time in the sun than adults do and dismiss health warnings as something that doesn't concern their immediate future. A skin cancer is for older people, they believe. The media doesn't help the cause either. Celebrities and supermodels proudly exhibit a seamless tan.

There are signs, however, that those sun-smart campaigns are slowly changing the behaviour. Sunscreens and even hats become essential items for some, but not all, sun worshippers. Nevertheless, the rapid growth of the melanoma rate has slowed in many countries.

Sun avoidance

Stay out of the sun and you won't have any problems. That's like suggesting not driving the car so you won't have any accidents, or don't eat fruit because they are full of insecticides—all over-the-top statements. No one wants you to hide in a dark cave. Too little sunshine is as unhealthy as overexposure is.

UV radiation is most damaging when the rays strike a surface at a right angle. You receive most radiation during summer around noon when the sun is high in the sky, so if you can avoid the two hours before and after the sun's zenith you drastically reduce the daily dose. This is particularly true at or near reflective surfaces such as water, sand and snow. The reflected UV rays are still strong enough to give you sunburn even in the shade, but burning takes up to twice as long.

Have you ever noticed how quiet nature becomes during a hot summer day? The animals are clever enough to have a siesta during the scorching midday hours. It is beyond my comprehension why organizers of sport or other activities schedule events during times of highest UV radiation—not to forget the health hazards of extreme heat that then come into play.

Tanning Devices

Sun beds, sun lamps, tanning beds, solariums et al are artificial tanning devices that emit high doses of mainly UVA light. UVA radiation is no longer considered safe—on the contrary. UVA light penetrates deeper into the skin than UVB light does and can equally damage or alter cell structures. Some devices emit several times more radiation than the sun does. Because damage accumulates, artificial UV radiation adds to sun exposure, so avoid tanning devices.

Antioxidants

During UV radiation bombardments, some cell molecules quite often lose some of their components. These molecules, named free radicals, are then competing with neighbouring molecules for 'spare parts.' The neighbours, however, may be a vital protein or DNA and can easily be damaged by the marauding free radicals—they oxidize.

A diet rich in antioxidants provides the free radicals with willing donors. Antioxidants in food sources such as fruit and vegetables, or in green tea and vitamin supplements, should reduce the risk of UV radiation damage. So far, however, the research is inconclusive.

Protection

'SLIP, SLOP, SLAP—slip on a shirt, slop on sunscreen, and slap on a hat.' This is the simple message anti-cancer organizations convey to potential sun seekers, especially children, in the hope that protection from UV radiation will reduce the number of skin cancer victims. Other organizations also advocate the wearing of appropriate clothing, sunglasses and sunscreens. But what is appropriate?

Clothing and sunglasses

Broad-rimmed hats provide the best protection for all parts of the head. Unfortunately, many people see this type of hat as not very fashionable, particularly men. Baseball caps are popular instead. But while shading the face, they don't protect ears and neck. Legionnaire hats are similar to baseball caps but have a flap in the back that protects the neck and to some degree the sides of the head.

Light-coloured and loose-fitting garments provide ideal protection and comfort in the sun. UV radiation does penetrate fabric, though. The amount of radiation reaching the skin depends largely on its weave. The denser the weave, the less UV radiation can pass through the fabric. Today some manufacturers of recreational clothing offer garments made of treated fabrics, which can triple the blocking capacity.

The public does seem to hear the message to protect the eyes against UV radiation. Hats are not in vogue everywhere, but luckily sunglasses are. It doesn't have to be the dark-tinted variety, as the darkness of the lenses only reduces glare. Treated clear prescription glasses and contact lenses can equally absorb UV radiation. Special sunglasses and goggles are available for certain sport and work activities.

Sunscreens

Of course, you don't want to enjoy the beach dressed like a mummy. Showing some flesh is part of the fun. Correctly used sunscreen can effectively protect those exposed body parts from harmful UV radiation. There is a catch: sunscreens only prolong the time before the skin is harmed. They may encourage people to stay in the sun longer, thus eliminating the benefits.

Sunscreen either absorbs, scatters or reflects UV radiation. Manufacturers advise the buyer on how well this process will work in their sunscreen. In most countries they are required by law to advertise the internationally accepted sun protection factor (SPF) for their product. The figure gives you an indication of how much longer you can stay in the sun before you get sunburn. For example, if you generally burn in 30 minutes without sunscreen, a product with a SPF rating of 15 should prolong the onset by a factor of 15, that is 7.5 hours.

Read the bottle's instruction in fine print. This factor is only valid if you apply enough sunscreen and reapply it regularly. Because sunscreen is not cheap, most people don't apply the required amount. Also, use a broad-spectrum sunscreen. This will protect you against UVA and UVB radiation.

Chapter Seven

Violent Weather

Blame violent weather for:

- Injury
- Death
- Destruction
- Diseases

and more

Introduction

Isn't this Toto, your neighbour's terrier floating past your bedroom window with its ears flapping? Oh boy, Dorothy is still holding onto the leash. Looks like a hell of a storm out there.

Days with destructive winds, lightning and floods are the times when 'Mother Nature' shows her bad temper. In a matter of minutes, her fury flattens whole neighbourhoods, towns or regions. Millions lose their homes and belongings every year. Some lose more than their possessions. Violent weather takes away the lives of thousands worldwide. Hurricane Mitch alone was responsible for the death of over 10,000 Hondurans in 1998.

On the average, about 50 Australians and over 1,000 US citizens die every year as a direct consequence of extreme weather events. The figure is likely to be much higher, however, because the cause of death is not always easily attributed to weather events.

The economic impact of destructive winds is, to some degree, more tangible. When a tornado or a cyclone ravages a town, an assessor estimates the replacement cost of homes and contents and the damage to the town's infrastructure. Not quite as easy is the assessment of secondary impacts, such as the temporary provision of shelter and food, long-term revenue shortfalls, reduced business activity etc.

Canada had a disastrous year in 1996. Violent weather caused more than A$5 billion worth of damage. Secondary impacts were estimated to exceed A$6 billion. More recent weather events are directly responsible for annual economic losses of over A$30 billion in the US. The figure does not include the significant impact of extreme heat or cold.

Transport is usually the first to suffer. A tropical cyclone or tornado warning stops public transport. The ensuing loss of revenue and possible accidents can reach several million dollars. Rain, snow and ice on roads cause fatalities and injuries every year. Insurance companies receive thousands of weather-related car insurance claims. Whether you are on a small pleasure craft or a large ferry, being on sea during violent storms is asking for trouble. Mountainous waves may capsize a seagoing vessel of almost any size.

No other transport system is as dependent on weather as aviation. Strong winds, turbulence, reduced visibility, icing, snow etc. cause cancellations or diversion of flights. The Air Transport Association estimates an annual weather-related loss of revenue of around A$540 million for its 26 member airlines.

The weather is never perfect for farmers. Too much rain and the soil washes away or the crops rot; not enough rain and the plants wilt. Hail damages the plants and makes fruit and vegetables non-saleable. Strong winds flatten the crops. The US vegetable processing industry estimates a weather-related loss of over A$80 million per year. You are not a farmer? You still have to pay, though, as the market prices skyrocket after natural disasters.

While we talk prices, violent weather dictates the amount of money you pay for your property insurance. That is, if you can get a policy. You probably won't go far with your application if you live in a flood-prone area. Alternatively, the insurance premium is very high in areas with high incidences of extreme weather events, e.g. floods, cyclones or tornadoes. Several billion dollars worth of damage comes quite naturally to a good-sized tropical cyclone.

You still aren't off the hook. As a taxpayer, you support the victims of disasters. Several government emergency agencies provide one-off payments or loans to their own citizens or to the people in disaster areas of other countries. In the long term, governments spend large amounts rebuilding damaged roads and public buildings.

What does the future hold? The insurance companies bet on massive increases in weather-related catastrophes. They cite two reasons: population growth and global warming. Popular waterfront areas, such as the southeast coast of the US or the northeast coast of Australia, have grown rapidly in population and will continue to grow. Emergency agencies and insurance companies know that one day a 'big one' will hit a major town, causing immense damage. Scientists claim that global warming will multiply and intensify extreme weather events.

WIND

What is wind?

Wind stirs your emotions. A gentle breeze feels good, especially on a hot day. When the wind picks up and dust or sand blows into your face, it becomes annoying. A warm dry mountain wind gets on your nerves and makes you feel sick. When the wind grows even stronger—tree branches break, roof tiles blow away—it becomes frightening.

Wind is very useful. For thousands of years, mankind used the wind to sail the oceans. Windmills ground the wheat or created electric power. Aircraft like the wind on their noses for short take-offs or landings. Wind disseminates plant seeds and pollen.

Wind is cruel, too. It causes considerable damage, injury and death: ships sink, aircraft crash, buildings collapse. A tornado needs only a few minutes to flatten your home, a cyclone threatens many kilometres of coastline, while winter storms bring traffic to a halt.

What drives the wind?

Wind creation

Wind is movement of the air. When you and I talk of wind we consider only the horizontal movement. Air moves three-dimensionally, though. To differentiate, the non-horizontal components have other names, such as updraughts, downdraughts, thermals, turbulence, etc.

It is the vertical movement that triggers the wind. Let's go to the supermarket car park on a hot summer's day. The sun heats up the bitumen and the parked cars. The hot surface and vehicles pass on some of the heat to the air just above it. The warm air near the car park's surface is less dense. It is, therefore, lighter than the slightly cooler air above it and rises. But unless the air is replenished, you would step into a vacuum when you walk to your car. This won't happen, of course. The car park draws fresh air from somewhere. But from where?

Coincidentally, there is a playground nearby. The local council spent a considerable amount of money to plant nice green grass and many leafy trees. The air is much cooler on the playground than it is on the car park. The air won't rise. Instead it has to move sideways to fill the 'hole' in the air above the car park. The movement is wind.

'Stop right here,' you say. 'Now the playground is without air.' Almost true. The playground has to supply all the rising air of the

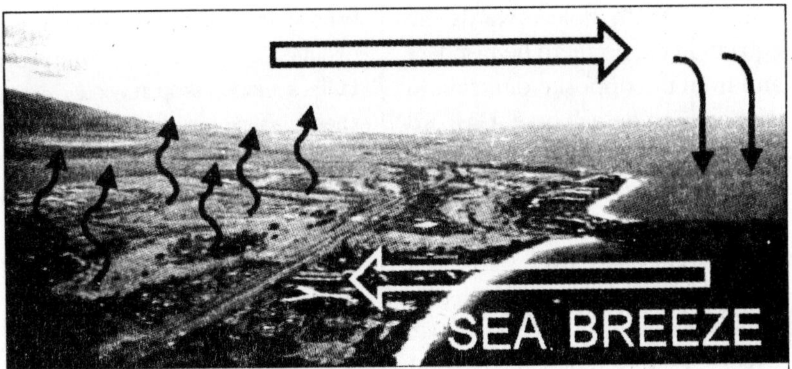

The warm air above the land rises and draws the cooler air from the sea. The upper air above the land travels towards the sea, cools down and descends to the sea's surface.

surrounding car park. Well, this rising air has to go somewhere. The upper layers of the atmosphere would be rather crowded with air if they couldn't shed some of it. By the laws of physics, rising air cools. It cools enough to allow some of it to descend in a downdraught and replenish the air on the playground. Nature created a loop, better known as air circulation.

In other words, warm air rises in an *updraught* until it cools enough to travel as *upper wind* to a position where it can descend in a *down-draught*. Once the air reaches the surface, it moves as *surface wind* to the place where the updraughts occurred.

The sea breeze is another welcome example of this process. The hot air above land rises and draws the soothing breeze from the ocean. On a larger scale, the same happens globally. The tropics provide the rising warm air and the poles the cool descent points. In between you have the prevailing winds.

If this is true, then the prevailing winds should be blowing directly from the North Pole towards the equator in the northern hemisphere and from the opposite direction in the southern hemisphere. Gaspard Coriolis (1792–1843), a French mathematician, had the same thought. He searched for an answer and discovered the deflecting forces of the earth's rotation—the Coriolis force.

Let's assume that you fly from Adelaide to Darwin, which is almost due north; you are not subject to wind influences; you do not follow navigational aids on

Wind talk

Sea breeze – during the day warm air rises over land and draws cooler air from the sea.

Land breeze – at night the sea is warmer than the land. Rising air over the sea draws the air from the land.

Gust – a sudden increase in wind speed, lasting only a few seconds.

Squall – a sudden increase in wind speed, lasting several minutes.

Lull – a sudden drop in wind speed, lasting only a few seconds.

Jet stream – a narrow band of strong winds above 10 km reaching speeds of up to 400 km/h.

Clear air turbulence – sudden up or downdraughts generally above 6 km. Occurs in 'clear' air, i.e. outside of clouds. Dreaded by airline passengers.

the way, and you are totally unaware of Gaspard's discovery. In such a scenario you could not travel in a straight line. While you are on your journey, the earth rotates underneath you and Darwin has moved some distance to the east. Your path as plotted onto the surface looks more like a hook. You will travel the last few kilometres almost west to east to catch up with Darwin. Highly trained airline pilots compensate for this fact. The wind lacks pilot training and doesn't compensate for the Coriolis effect. Most prevailing winds on earth are, therefore, blowing from west to east. There are always exceptions, of course.

The next time you sit in your bath tub or spa bath, you can become your own discoverer. There are a lot of things to explore in the bath, but when you pull the plug you will observe that the water drains in a rotating funnel-like manner—just like looking into a tornado or a tropical cyclone from above. It's no coincidence—the same force that makes your draining bath water spin also acts on tornadoes, hurricanes, low-pressure systems, dust devils etc.

When you watch the weather forecast on television you see low (L) and high (H) pressure systems marked on the map. They are also the products of unequal temperatures on the earth's surface. An area with low density and rising air has less air pressure than the neighbouring area with cool and descending air. Wind spirals from 'High' to 'Low.'

The winds between the two pressure systems are often so strong that they override local air movements, in which case your car park doesn't develop its own wind pattern and the sea breeze is non-existent or delayed.

How is wind measured?

When I tell you that my town was buffeted by strong winds yesterday, you want to know how strong the wind was. Without comparable figures, the word 'strong' is almost meaningless. It depends on how a person perceives a strong wind—it is subjective.

In the absence of instruments, early seafarers relied on accurate descriptions of wind strength. In 1806, Admiral Sir Francis Beaufort of the Royal Navy devised a scale and attributed numbers to the state of the sea. For example, very light air movement results in a few ripples on the water's surface—he named it strength 1. Only a strong breeze manages to spray water off the top of the waves—strength 6. Wind strengths of between 12 and 17 describe the different categories of tropical cyclones. The scale was so successful that observers on land adapted it to their needs. The description of the wind is still in use today.

The Beaufort Scale wasn't accurate enough for modern usage. Unfortunately, when the time came to look for a replacement, the world couldn't agree on one system. The following methods of measuring wind speed are now in use worldwide:

- **Nautical miles per hour**, known as **knots** (kt), also measures a ship's or aircraft's speed. 1 kt = 1.85 km/h, 1.15 mph
- **Statute miles per hour** (mph), imperial unit. 1 mph = 1.61 km/h
- **Kilometres per hour** (km/h), metric unit. 1 km/h = 0.62 mph
- **Meters per second** (mps, m/sec), metric unit, measures horizontal and vertical air movements. 1 m/sec = 3.3 ft/sec
- **Feet per minute** (ft/min), is only used to measure vertical air movements. Commonly used in aviation to indicate an aircraft's descent and climb.
- **Beaufort Scale**, ranges from 0–17 and indicates the force of the wind.

The wind is generally stronger the higher up it is, because the friction of trees and buildings slows it near the surface. To compare wind speeds, weather services around the world have agreed to place their wind speed measuring device 10 m above the ground.

To indicate the wind direction, only two scales are in use: the 32 compass points (north, south, southwest etc.) and the 360° of a circle. When you use a compass as a navigation device you point it towards the direction you want to walk or drive—e.g. east or north, 90° or 360°. To indicate the wind direction, however, the observer measures the direction from where the wind comes from. In other words, a wind that blows in a southern direction is a northerly wind. It comes from the north and you are looking north when the wind blows into your face.

The Beaufort Scale

Beaufort number	Description	Wind speed mph	km/h	knots	Observations
0	Calm	0	0	0	Tree leaves don't move, smoke rises vertically.
1	Light air	1–3	1–5	1–3	Tree leaves don't move, smoke drifts slowly.
2	Light breeze	4–7	6–11	4–6	Tree leaves rustle, flags wave slightly, wind felt on face, weather vane is active.
3	Gentle breeze	8–11	12–19	7–10	Leaves and twigs move, light flags extended.
4	Moderate breeze	13–18	20–29	11–16	Small branches move, flags flap, dust and paper drift.
5	Fresh breeze	19–24	30–38	17–27	Small trees sway, flags flap and ripple.
6	Strong breeze	25–31	39–50	22–27	Large branches sway, flags beat and pop, umbrellas difficult to use.
7	Moderate gale	32–38	51–61	28–33	Whole trees sway, difficult to walk against wind.
8	Fresh gale	39–46	62–85	34–40	Twigs break off trees, walking becomes very difficult.
9	Strong gale	47–54	75–86	41–47	Branches break off trees, tiles blown from roofs, slight damage to buildings.
10	Whole gale	55–63	87–101	48–55	Some trees uprooted, damage to buildings.
11	Storm	64–74	102–120	56–63	Widespread damage.
12–17	Hurricane	>75	>120	>64	Severe and extensive damage. Six categories.

Thunderstorms

Evolution of a thunderstorm

When you hear thunder, you have a thunderstorm nearby. As obvious as it sounds, that is the definition of a thunderstorm: no thunder—no thunderstorm. If only everything else were so simple. Mind you, the weather services came up with some conditions. For example, you must have heard the thunder within the last 10-15 minutes. Now it's official.

Ever wondered how far away the thunderstorm is? Because light travels faster than sound does, you can determine the distance by counting the seconds between a lightning flash and the arrival of its associated thunderclap. A difference of three seconds represents approximately one kilometre.

How does a thunderstorm develop? There are several ways, but generally it requires air to lift, to cool and water vapour to condense.

The most common type is the afternoon *heat thunderstorm*. Remember the hot car park? A heated surface warms the air above it. The air rises and cools in the process. At a certain temperature (dew point) the water vapour condenses and forms a tiny puffy cloud (cumulus). If the conditions are right, the cloud continuous to grow until it hits an invisible ceiling—the tropopause, a layer that heats up with height and forms a strong inversion (see Chapter Three, 'Air'). When the rising air in the growing cloud reaches this layer, it will have the same temperature as the tropopause and stop moving upward. As a consequence, the cloud spreads underneath the inversion and forms the characteristic anvil of a cumulonimbus cloud. The flat top is above the freezing level where water droplets freeze. The ice crystals give the cloud's top a feathery and ragged look.

Conditions for thunderstorm development

- **Instability.** The atmosphere must be unstable, i.e. no temperature inversions between the surface and the tropopause.
- **Humidity.** Enough water vapour must be present to supply the demand of a cumulonimbus cloud.
- **Trigger mechanism.** Air has to rise in order to form a convective cloud. The trigger can be a warm surface, a mountain range or a weather front.

Forced lifting creates other types of thunderstorm. When air is forced up the slopes of a mountain range the same process begins and an *orographic thunderstorm* develops. Cold air masses from polar regions wedge underneath warmer air and force it upwards. This is the characteristic of a cold front, and if thunderstorms develop along the front they are named *frontal thunderstorms.*

A cumulonimbus cloud contains very strong updraughts and turbulence. Water droplets and ice crystals collide and form rain, hail or snow (precipitation). The strong updraughts keep the precipitation within the cloud until it becomes too heavy. Then the heavy water droplets, ice balls or snowflakes fall out of the cloud. The weatherman calls this a shower.

This is also the end in the life cycle of a thunderstorm. The falling precipitation creates heavy downdraughts. They overpower the updraughts eventually and dry out the cloud from the top. In addition, the surface is now wet and cool and no longer able to supply the cloud with warm air. The thunderstorm dies.

Observation and lightning detectors give the weatherman a good idea where the thunderstorms occur, how many there are at any given moment and in which direction they are drifting. Nevertheless, forecasting a heat thunderstorm is a thankless task. The meteorologist knows when the conditions for the development are favourable and predicts thunderstorms for the next day. But ask the forecaster whether your town will get one and he may answer, 'Beats me.'

Thunderstorm hazards

A country the size of the US or Australia experiences approximately 10,000 thunderstorms each year. Most of the time, they are nothing but a nuisance. From a distance, you may even enjoy the spectacular cumulonimbus cloud and the bonus 'fireworks' of lightning and thunder. Occasionally, however, a severe thunderstorm can be as destructive as a tropical cyclone or a tornado. A single severe thunderstorm unleashes its fury over an area of about 8 km. Sometimes, especially along a weather front, thunderstorms come in company and line up for more than 150 km.

Annually, their destructive power results in economic losses in the US of around A$2 billion. In Australia, thunderstorms are more damaging than cyclones, floods or bushfires. Of course, there are exceptional years when the competition takes first place.

Thunderstorms just about have it all. They present you with a variety of hazards and all are potentially destructive. Amongst them are:

- **Strong winds** inflict the first damage. Severe thunderstorms deal out gusts exceeding 80 km/h, often before the cloud arrives. In 1991 a thunderstorm crossed the North Shore of Sydney, Australia, with wind gusts of up to 230 km/h, causing injury to 100 people and leaving a damage bill of around A$680 million. The storm damaged 10,000 buildings and in excess of 50,000 trees.
- Vertical air movement just underneath the cloud can produce even stronger gusts. **Downbursts** or **microbursts**, the term depends on the size of the outflow, quite often result in gusts of up to 240 km/h. Mention microburst in the presence of an airline pilot and you see a sudden change in his or her facial expression. An aircraft, large or small, is very vulnerable to shifts in wind speed and direction during take-off or landing—a 'sitting duck' so to speak. Microbursts are strong enough to drive an aircraft into the ground and have been the cause of several major accidents.
- Strong updraughts keep **hailstones** within the cloud where they grow until they are heavy enough to overcome the vertical air movement. Hail causes major damage to agricultural crops every year. Occasionally, the hailstones can reach a size that damages buildings and cars. Sydney was again the target of a severe weather event in 1999: hailstones the size of tennis balls damaged 22,000 homes and 63,000 cars. Even aircraft at the international airport weren't spared. The insurance companies claim that the total damage bill exceeded A$2.3 billion.
- **Flash floods.** Thunderstorms can dump an immense amount of rain on a small area. The soil is soon soaked and the drainage system is incapable of removing the excess water. Dangerous flash floods develop very quickly and are potential killers.
- **Lightning** kills and injures people. People usually underestimate the danger of lightning because it selects its victims at random. You think it's very unlucky to be struck by lightning? Not so. The odds are much shorter than winning the major prize in a lotto game. Lightning is also a major cause of bushfires.
- Severe thunderstorms occasionally develop **tornadoes**. The destructive winds in the narrow funnel destroy everything in its path. See the following section for more information.

Tornadoes

A tornado is a revolving column of air in a funnel-shaped cloud extending from the base of a cumulonimbus (thunderstorm cloud) to the ground. The entry to the funnel is only a few hundred metres wide but contains destructive winds with speeds exceeding 320 km/h. The same phenomenon over water is called a waterspout.

During the mature stage of a severe thunderstorm, very strong updraughts feed parts of the insatiable cumulonimbus cloud. In other parts of the cloud, severe downdraughts occur. It is in this extremely turbulent region, between rising and descending air, where tornadoes are born. If the conditions are right, the turbulence becomes organized and the air starts to spin, just like the draining water in the bathtub. The rotation is very unstable and may last only a few minutes, long enough to cause immense damage on the ground.

Occasionally tornadoes form underneath tropical thunderstorms in cyclones. Severe thunderstorms with tornadoes are more frequent in the mid-latitudes, however, where air masses with significant temperature differences clash. The intensity of the clash increases when a region has mountain ranges funnelling either air mass towards its adversary. The US has such mountain ranges. Warm and humid air from the Gulf of Mexico meets with cold Canadian air over the Central States, known as 'Tornado Alley'.

While tornadoes occur worldwide, the US holds the record with 1,297 in one year (1992). Australia is second with several hundreds per year, but a sparse population prevents an accurate count. The plains of China and Argentina are also a favourite breeding ground for tornadoes. Waterspouts frequently cross the coast and develop into tornadoes in many coastal and island nations.

Despite their destructive powers, tornadoes don't account for many deaths. Floods and even lightning cause a higher mortality rate. Nevertheless, approximately 100 US citizens die and about twenty times as many get injured every year. The economic losses are tremendous, though. Every year is different, but the damage is generally somewhere between A$800 million to over A$2 billion in the US. Because tornadoes accompany severe thunderstorms, hail and flood damage usually add to the figures.

Unless the tornado strikes buildings, farmers don't usually suffer great losses. The tornado destroys everything within its narrow path, but has minimal impact on the rest of the crop. The wind damage is high in built-up areas where it cuts a swath of destruction. The destructive path can be so selective that one house gets completely demolished while the other next to it remains untouched. The type of building also influences the severity of the damage. Pre-fabricated housing and mobile homes suffer most.

Tornadoes strike without warning—almost. The weather forecasters know when severe thunderstorms are likely to develop and, because tornadoes come with severe thunderstorms, they can issue a tornado watch. Some weather stations are equipped with radar capable of detecting air in motion. Observed rotating air within the thunderstorm or actual witnessed tornadoes by weather service personnel or the public activate a tornado warning. Unfortunately, communities near the thunderstorm don't have much time to react.

Tropical cyclones

'Tropical cyclone' is the general term for an intense low-pressure system in the tropics. Its features are revolving storms and cloud bands around a centre of very low atmospheric pressure. In the Americas its name is *hurricane*, in Asia *typhoon* and in Australia simply *cyclone*.

Tropical cyclones develop from low-pressure systems. Warm and moist air lifts over a large area and draws air from the surroundings, creating wind. The deflection of the earth's rotation, the Coriolis effect, forces the wind to rotate around the calm centre. A circle of severe

Tropical cyclone categories

Category	Description	Wind speed			
		m/s	km/h	mph	knots
1	weak	33-42	118-153	73-95	64-82
2	moderate	43-49	154-177	96-110	83-96
3	strong	50-58	178-209	111-130	97-113
4	very strong	59-70	210-250	131-155	114-135
5	destructive	>70	>250	>155	>135

thunderstorms forms and draws an ever-increasing amount of air. The air pressure in the centre falls steadily. If the conditions are right, the system becomes self-generating. Finally, when the wind speed exceeds 118 km/h, a tropical cyclone is born.

A mature tropical cyclone shows a distinct cloudless eye, surrounded by very strong winds and bands of severe thunderstorms. The system remains alive until it moves over a region with lower water temperatures or over land. In either case, the supply of warm and moist air stops. Before it dies, however, the system dumps a large amount of rain and may cause widespread flooding.

Weather services around the world agree on one particular scale to categorize tropical cyclones. This scale, the Saffir-Simpson scale, uses five wind speed ranges as indicators of a cyclone's power.

Satellites, weather radar and reconnaissance flights allow the meteorologist to keep track of a tropical cyclone. The difficult part is to predict its next move. Cyclone movements are very erratic and sometimes they don't move at all. The strength varies constantly and even a 'dead' cyclone may come back to life. The forecaster has no option other than warning the population of a large section of coastline. A large percentage of the population is, therefore, only moderately affected by the storm and may become complacent the next time.

Will a global climate change bring us more and stronger tropical cyclones? Very likely. Scientists estimate that a small water temperature rise of less than one degree could extend the cyclone season by 20 days. Tropical cyclones need water temperatures of at least 26.5°C to develop and survive, so rising water temperatures will expand the area of activity. The Americas have another reason to fear imminent bad seasons. Caribbean hurricanes follow a 20-year cycle of changing activity levels. US meteorologists warn that the hurricanes are entering a phase of increased activity.

Tropical cyclone damage

Don't you long for a house on a beach with a million-dollar view? From your observation deck you can see the kids and the dog play in the azure waters of the tropical ocean. No more shivering in winter blizzards. All you need to wear is, well—not much at all. Oh, and don't forget—the nearest neighbour is kilometres away.

The dream becomes increasingly real for millions of people—at least part of it. Around 83% of the Australian population live within 50 km of the coastline (1996 census). The US expects 73 million people will make the coastline and a warm climate their home by the year 2010. But you don't have to look to the future for population growth. Tropical Queensland is the fastest growing state in Australia. And between 1988 and 1993, the population of Florida increased by more than one third. This, of course, shatters the dream of a secluded lifestyle.

The population growth along the coast ensures an ever-increasing damage bill. If the predictions of increased cyclone activity due to global warming hold true, you don't have to be a seer to predict a 'big' one.

A tropical cyclone causes damage in three ways:

1. Flood

Rising water levels and large waves are the heralds of worse to come. Low atmospheric pressure in the centre of the cyclone raises the sea level, as if it were 'sucking up' the ocean. The rise can be anything up to 1.5 m. In addition, strong winds around the eye pound the seas and whip up mountainous waves.

If the raised water and the waves reach the shallows of the coast and encounter a sloping beach, they grow even higher. And if this combination, called a storm surge, is trapped in a bay, the sea level can gain the height of a two-storey building: around 5 m. Many major harbour cities are well below this mark. Some are even below mean sea level, only protected by embankments.

In 1969, the 'ifs' came together in the Bay of Bengal and caused the worst weather-related disaster in history. Over 250,000 citizens of Bangladesh lost their lives. The 1900 storm surge ahead of an unnamed hurricane that swept across Galveston, US, killed more than 8,000 people, and showed that water can be more devastating than wind.

These situations are rare, but even waves half the size that last several hours can cause enough trouble. Then you find out if your builder has done a good job on your house's foundations: will it still stand after all the sand or soil has been washed away, or will it float like a boat and be driven away by strong winds?

2. Wind

Very strong winds, sometimes lasting for several hours, blow across communities, causing immense damage to housing and infrastructure. While the wind doesn't exact a high death toll—the average annual death toll from hurricanes in the US is below 100—the economic costs can reach many billions of dollars.

When hurricane Hugo struck South Carolina in 1989, it left a damage bill of almost A$20 billion. Three years later, in 1992, hurricane Andrew surpassed this mark with damage to insured properties in excess of A$30 billion. Experts believe that the bill is likely more than double the amount if they could add the uncalculated damage to uninsured properties.

Several cyclones cross the Australian coast every year. In 1974, tropical cyclone Tracy destroyed Darwin with winds of up to 250 km/h. Of 11,200 homes, only 400 remained in reasonable condition. To avoid an outbreak of diseases, over 35,000 residents were evacuated. The cyclone killed 65 people.

The winds of a tropical cyclone are generally not quite as strong as the swirling air inside a tornado, but size is an issue. Tropical cyclones are often over 500 km in diameter. Large storms in the Philippines and Japan occasionally reach a size of 1,600 km. The zone of destructive winds, sometimes in excess of 250 km/h, covers an area of over 50 km. If this isn't bad enough, the system also takes its time. The destructive winds can blow for several hours before they pass a particular point. The tropical cyclone itself may last for a week or more.

The wind itself is often only indirectly responsible for building collapses. Windborne debris, such as tree branches, roof tiles, metal sheeting etc. destroy roofs, windows and walls. Strong winds can then go to work and disassemble the rest. Flying debris inflicted most damage to homes in Darwin when tropical cyclone Tracy hit the town.

3. Rain

Of course, a punctured roof or broken window can't keep out the third burden: rain. Quite often, the content of a factory or home is more valuable than the building itself. The building may withstand the fury of the wind, but the hole in the roof or the broken window is enough to destroy your million-dollar machinery or stamp collection.

A tropical cyclone carries a large amount of moisture in the cloud bands around the eye. In 1998, hurricane Mitch devastated communities in Central America, in particular Honduras. Torrential rain caused heavy local floods (flash floods), river floods and mud slides, which killed more than 10,000 Hondurans, left several million people homeless and destroyed the economies of struggling nations.

Non-tropical cyclones

If the experts name a weather phenomenon tropical cyclone, then logic implies that there should be a non-tropical cyclone. There is, although the weatherman on your TV is more likely to call it a low-pressure system. In mid-latitudes, where tropical and polar air constantly battle for supremacy, low-pressure systems develop frequently. During winter and spring, such systems, with their warm and cold fronts, may pass over your town several times per week. Occasionally a system is strong enough to resemble a tropical cyclone.

In 1996, a Pacific storm lashed the West Coast of Canada, causing an estimated A$400 million dollars worth of damage. One hundred and fifty thousand homes were without power, and others collapsed under the weight of heavy snow. Five hundred avalanches were reported. Central Europe received an unwanted Christmas present in 1999 when a similar system created havoc. Orly airport in Paris recorded wind gusts of up to 173 km/h. The storm toppled 140,000 trees around Paris and 60 people were reported to have lost their lives across Europe.

LIGHTNING

A giant anvil-shaped cloud hovers above the ocean on a hot summer evening. An orange setting sun illuminates the feathery top of the cumulonimbus, while the rest is shrouded in darkness. But now and then the whole cloud glows bluish white and streaks of lightning flicker between the cloud and the water. Thunder rolls towards the shore. The display is a spectacular show, rivalling the New Year's Eve fireworks. It is also very dangerous.

A family of three enjoys their evening walk along a popular beach. They walk close to each other without holding hands. A lightning bolt strikes the mother who walks in-between her husband and her son. The mother dies instantly. The rest of the family doesn't receive a scratch, apart from the emotional scars.

The ancient Greeks would have said that Zeus was angry with the woman for whatever reason and tossed one of his golden thunderbolts towards her. If the woman had survived the 200 million-volt experience, she either must have possessed mythic powers or was protected by a rival god.

Today we know that Zeus must have been very busy in his time, because lightning is not a rare event. The US Lightning Detection Network registers over 20 million earth-bound lightning flashes per year. Worldwide, approximately 860,000 lightning flashes occur each day and during the time it takes for you to blink, several thousand lightning bolts strike the ground or water somewhere. Lightning is a frequent and random weather phenomenon.

The weather services can't predict where lightning will strike. But they can warn whenever thunderstorms are likely to develop. Then it is up to you to take the appropriate precautions.

What is lightning?

The *Oxford Dictionary* defines lightning as: '. . . the occurrence of a natural electrical discharge of very short duration and high voltage between a cloud and the ground or within a cloud, accompanied by a bright flash and typically also thunder.'

How does lightning form? Scientists aren't very sure, but support one popular theory. Strong turbulence within a thunderstorm cloud forces raindrops and ice crystals to collide. The drops and crystals stick together and grow bigger. They can't always sustain their size in the turbulent air and often split again into smaller fragments of unequal size. Experiments show different charges in the fragments. The smaller pieces are negatively charged whereas the larger pieces are positively charged. Updraughts and downdraughts take the fragments to different parts of the cloud, thus creating an imbalance of electrical charge within the cloud and between the cloud and the ground. Sparks will fly, literally, when the opposing forces are able to overcome the insulating property of the air. And what sparks they are. A lightning flash is the result of around 200 million volts' potential difference, and discharges in a current of several thousands amperes.

Most lightning occurs within the clouds. Only about 20% strike the surface. Because air is a good insulator, the lightning tends to take the shortest route towards a high object on the surface or a path with least resistance. If you are on a boat with your new graphite fishing rod in your hand, you are likely to be the highest point and an ideal target for a strike—a lightning strike, that is.

With lightning comes thunder. A lightning bolt heats the air in its path to over 40,000°C, causing it to expand rapidly and send out a strong shock wave. Your ear receives the change in air pressure and registers it as a loud noise.

Lightning damage, injury and death

With population growth, lightning damage to property increases. The US National Weather Service (NWS) estimates an annual cost to US society of A$70 million. The National Lightning Safety Institute, however, takes into account the indirect costs of bushfires, power blackouts, aircraft mishaps, and estimates a damage bill of around A$10 billion per year.

Do you play lotto? The odds that your six numbers are drawn from the 49 tumbling balls is around one in 14 million. You have a much better chance to be hit by lightning—less than one in half a million.

The US weather service reports approximately 100 deaths and 500 injuries per year from lightning strikes but other agencies believe that, due to under-reporting, the number of fatalities should be around 450. Australia has up to 10 deaths and well over 100 injuries per year. Conservative estimates put the worldwide toll at 1,000 deaths and 5,000 injuries annually. This makes lightning deadlier than tornadoes.

Nevertheless, the numbers show that you won't necessarily die when you are hit by lightning. If you use the US figures, the mortality rate is 20%, whereas the Australian rate is 10% of all lightning hits. But some studies suggest that, due to frequent underreporting of lightning injuries, the rate should be below five per cent. In other words, the survival rate is very high.

When you imagine a strike, you probably picture a lightning bolt enter a person's head and leave via the feet—a *direct strike.* Of course, this is the most deadly form of lightning strikes. Eighty per cent of victims don't survive. Fortunately, direct strikes are rare.

More common are indirect hits. Lightning often seeks a prominent object on the ground such as a tower or tree. The current enters a person in contact with the object—*contact potential*—or arcs a short distance to a person nearby—*side flash.* Sometimes the current travels through the soil and enters the body parts in contact with the ground, *step voltage.* In all cases, the object or the ground takes the brunt of the energy and the person has a good chance of survival.

Metal is a good conductor of electricity. It is, therefore, no surprise that a person in contact with or in proximity of electric cables, water pipes, household appliances or the telephone can become a victim of a lightning strike—*surge propagation.* Death is rare, but injuries are relatively common, in particular while using the telephone.

Lightning doesn't leave your remains in a pile of smoking ashes. Cardiac arrest is the main cause of death. Quite often, though, the heart automatically begins to beat again, but lack of oxygen, caused by a paralysed breathing mechanism, may stop the heart for a second time. A direct hit often causes horrific burns or scalding from evaporating moisture on the skin and in the lungs. In most cases, however, the human body acts like the shell of a car. The current flashes along the outside into the ground. Like the metal exterior of a car, the skin of a human protects its contents. In this case, survivors sometimes have no physical problems and clinical tests show normal results. They may see their physician with other serious after-effects, though.

Lightning injuries are different from household or industrial electric shocks and often misunderstood by the medical profession. Specialists in *keraunomedicine* study the effects of lightning strikes. Some of the known injuries and long-term effects are:

- External and internal burns and scalding
- Chronic pain
- Severe headache
- Severe ear damage, hearing loss, tinnitus

- Stiffness in joints, muscle spasm, numbness
- Sleep disturbance
- Memory loss, attention deficit
- Depression, inability to cope, irritability
- Dizziness, coordination problems, confusion
- General weakness, chronic fatigue
- Reduced libido
- Phobias.

Lightning safety

If you are a young man and play sport on an open field on a weekend afternoon in summer, you are asking for trouble. According to US lightning statistics published by the National Oceanic and Atmospheric Administration, men are four times more likely to be struck by lightning than women are. They tend to spend more time outdoors when thunderstorms develop—summer afternoons.

No matter what your gender is, you can further increase the risk in other ways. Being at or near a tall object, or being the tall object yourself, is risky. People often take shelter under a tree to avoid a shower of rain. Trees are not very good conductors of electricity, though. A lightning bolt may leave the tree trunk and continue the journey via an unsuspecting person. Metal towers are good conductors, but in this case, the ground underneath a person's feet is heavily charged with electricity—not a good place to be.

You also shouldn't be on a hill enjoying the spectacle of a free lightning show. Lightning is in such a hurry to reach the ground that it often overlooks the value of a human being. It takes the shortest route—you. Water is a good conductor, too. Since there are no trees or towers on a lake or the ocean, the tallest object is undoubtedly your boat.

Any good conductor at or near your body increases the risk. Avoid using electric appliances or the telephone during thunderstorm activities. Standing on a moist ground is not a good idea either.

Lightning is random and, therefore, very unpredictable. You as an individual must take responsibility for yourself and persons in your care. All tips and safety measures are only designed to minimize the risk, not to provide absolute protection. Take the following precautions:

- **Listen to warnings.** While no forecaster can predict the place of a lightning impact, he or she can issue a warning that thunderstorms will occur in your region. This is the time to plan your activities accordingly.
- **Recognize the danger.** Large clouds extending high into the atmosphere with a dark and flat bottom and a feathery anvil-shaped top are most likely thunderstorm clouds (cumulonimbus). Soon you either see the first flashes or hear some distant rumbling. Estimate the distance by counting the time between a flash and the arrival of the thunder. For every kilometre the sound takes about three seconds to travel. This doesn't work if you have a serious of flashes and you can't associate a single flash with the arriving thunder. When the thunderstorm has passed, suspend all activity for another 30 minutes. Lightning may still be present in a dying thunderstorm. Statistics prove that the most dangerous times for lightning injuries are just before and at the apparent end of storms.
- **Seek shelter.** Electricity likes to flash around the outside of an object. With exceptions, of course, a car or a house provides good protection. Avoid shelter under trees or any other tall and free-standing structure.
- **Outdoors.** If you are the coordinator of an outdoor event, plan the evacuation and safety measures well in advance. Suspend activities when you see lightning or hear thunder. Whether you are a group or a single person, avoid high ground, open spaces, water, and metal objects. Definitely don't be the highest point in the surrounding space.
- **Indoors.** Lightning can enter your house via electric wiring, phone lines or water pipes. Do not use electric appliances and avoid phone calls. Don't take a bath or a shower.

Lightning victims don't carry a charge. They are safe to touch and most will survive when given immediate first aid. Call for professional help, then follow first aid procedures, such as evacuation from a high risk area and resuscitation if required.

By the way, if you still think that lightning never strikes twice, think again. On average, lightning strikes the Empire State Building in New York 23 times each year.

FLOODS

Did the ancient Hebrews breach international copyright laws by borrowing the story of Noah's flood from the Babylonian Gilgamesh epic? Obviously no such law existed in biblical times, but both stories have significant similarities. If you take the written words into consideration, the Babylonians were first. Jews and Christians argue, however, that their ancestors didn't write down everything that happened. So, who was the first to report the flood of 'biblical proportions'? I guess the question mark will stay forever.

Forty days and forty nights. That is how long Noah's flood supposedly lasted. American marine archaeologists and geologists claim the duration was more likely forty years. They found evidence that people inhabited the bottom of the Black Sea about 7,500 years ago, and speculate that rising waters in the Mediterranean broke through the narrow strip of land (today's Bosporus at Istanbul) and inundated the low-lying area. For the population of this area it must have felt like a flood that never stopped. Fortunately, modern floods don't last that long, but are nevertheless devastating.

Floods are a part of the natural processes that shape the earth. The regular floods of the mighty rivers on our planet provide whole ecosystems with moisture and soil fertility. River deltas are the richest agricultural areas on earth, and some of the largest cities are located on the flood plains.

To protect their citizens, government authorities try to manage the regularly occurring floods. Dams, levees and channels are some of the common measures of flood control. Very often, however, these measures amplify the negative effects of floods. For example, raised river banks protect land from the waters of a swollen river until the embankments break or overflow. Before embankments were built, flood waters would quickly recede to the river once its water level dropped. With embankments, however, the flood waters remain trapped in low-lying areas for many days or weeks. Straightening the natural flow of a river system and concreting its banks leads to an increase in the speed of its water flow, and otherwise tame rivers become torrents. Draining wetlands and replacing them with paved asphalt retards the absorption process, so that the runoffs cause flash floods.

The rainwater catchment areas are often in other countries and/or populated by people ignorant to the plight of their fellow humans downstream. Clear-felling the Himalaya slopes in India, for example, results in devastating floods in downstream Bangladesh. In addition, unsustainable farming practices and replacing natural vegetation with man-made structures increases the negative effects of floods.

Water can cause floods in several ways:

- **Rainfall.** Heavy rainfall, especially in the catchment areas, swells creeks and streams. These contributories feed the main rivers, resulting in major flooding downstream (river floods). Runoff rainwater from brief but intense thunderstorms causes local flooding (flash floods).
- **Storm surge.** The storms of tropical and non-tropical cyclones can raise the sea to flood levels, inundating low-lying coastal areas.
- **Global warming.** Scientists warn that global warming will melt some of the polar ice. A permanent rise of the ocean level will submerge many coastal communities and islands.
- **Tsunami.** Earth quakes and volcano eruptions can create mountainous waves that strike coasts and islands with immense force and speed. Depending on the geographical characteristics of a coastline, the tsunami can travel several kilometres inland.
- **Dams.** Natural or man-made landslides block the path of a river, causing flooding upstream. The ice of a frozen river cracks in spring and may collect in narrow passages, forming a temporary dam. When purpose-built dams fail, they spill their contents in a rush.

Death and destruction

Each cause is bad enough on its own. Sometimes factors combine, though, leading to an immense death toll and damage. The floods in Bangladesh are a typical example. Heavy monsoon rain on the deforested slopes of the Himalayas swell the Ganges to flood levels annually. If, at the same time, tropical storms raise the ocean level, the floods are likely to kill thousands and displace millions of people.

China suffered devastating flooding in 1998. Government authorities reported a death toll of 3,656 and the displacement of 14 million people. The floods caused over A$40 billion worth of damage. In 1999, floods across Asia killed more than 1,000 people. Around 1,140 mm of rain fell over Eastern Europe in 1997, killing 100, affecting more than one million people and costing over A$4 billion. Flash floods kill 146 people annually in the US, making it the number one weather-related killer.

Queensland, Australia, received record rainfalls in 1974 that caused major flooding in the state capital, Brisbane. The floods claimed the lives of 16 people and injured 300. The estimated damage was almost A$ 1 billion. In 1990, a flood covered more than one million square kilometres of inland New South Wales and Queensland—an area larger than the United Kingdom and France combined. The floodwaters drowned up to one million farm animals.

Diseases

Diseases follow the floods. Dislocated people seek refuge in makeshift shelters with no or inadequate sanitation, or on the last dry patches of earth where food and clean drinking water is scarce. High temperatures quickly breed infectious diseases in the foul floodwaters.

Some of the infectious diseases associated with floods are:

- **Gastroenteritis** is the non-specific term for the inflammation of the stomach. A variety of viruses can infect a person drinking floodwater or eating infected fish. Diarrhoea and vomiting are the main symptoms. Although generally not dangerous, the loss of fluids sometimes requires hospitalization.
- **Dysentery.** *Shigella* bacteria in floodwater contaminate drinking water and food. The organism is the main cause of epidemic dysentery, a serious form of diarrhoea. Up to 10% of reported cases worldwide are fatal, with children most at risk.
- **Typhoid.** Typhoid fever is an acute bacterial infection transmitted via contaminated water or food. The disease affects approximately 16 million people in developing countries. Basic hygiene practices are the main weapon against typhoid, but are difficult to apply during flood events.
- **Cholera** is another serious bacterial infection of the intestines. Severe diarrhoea and vomiting dehydrates the patient. The fatality rate is very high if medical attention is not readily available.
- **Giardiasis** is one of the most common parasitic infections following floods. The illness is a problem in all parts of the world. It shows itself most often in the form of diarrhoea, nausea and abdominal cramps, which can take several days to appear and last for up to six weeks.

- **Malaria.** Receding floodwater leaves vast breeding grounds for mosquitoes. When the immune system of flood victims is weakened by poor health, the mosquito-borne disease finds easy targets.

Floodwaters drive **rodents** and **snakes** out of their shelters and into dry homes or refugee camps. Rats and mice are hosts to many diseases and parasites, adding to the health hazards. The rodents and snakes are understandably in a panic and may show aggressive behaviour.

THE FUTURE

Dreaming of a white Christmas? Dream on. Snow-covered pine trees and horse-drawn sleds may become a thing of the past in many parts of the world. There is no denying it any more—global warming is real. Independent scientists and governments established that the world is around 0.6°C warmer this century. The European average annual temperature increased even more: 0.8°C.

This increase may not sound very alarming but even such slight increases can have significant consequences. In the last decade you have heard of record high temperatures, record floods and droughts, severe storms and a record number of tornadoes. Northern Europe is already measurably wetter and southern Europe drier than it was before the twentieth century. Icebergs the size of small countries break off the polar shelf ice and make the sea levels rise. European and US insurers have already had dramatic increases in payments over the past decade. The United States' insured losses have risen from A$3.2 billion in the 1980s to A$20 billion in the 1990s.

Ironically, some scientists warn that Europe may eventually become colder as a result of global warming. Europe enjoys relatively mild weather due to the Gulf Stream, a warm ocean current flowing from the Gulf of Mexico across the Atlantic to Europe. A slight increase of the ocean temperature in the polar region will melt some of the permanent ice and end up diverting the Gulf Stream away from the European coast. Europe could then expect similar severe annual cold snaps similar to those in Canada and the US.

Biometeorological researchers probably don't care much about the snow at Christmas. They are more concerned about the long-term effect that global warming and ozone layer depletion has on people and on the environment. They expect an increase in extreme weather events, which means more people will suffer or die. More heat waves, severe floods, mudslides and storms may become the norm rather than the exception. More people will be displaced permanently or temporarily because of climatic changes.

The World Health Organization warns of indirect consequences of global warming, and most scientists agree on the following impacts:

- Greater number of severe heat waves and weather extremes
- More floods and droughts

- The regional distribution of infectious diseases and its carriers will change
- Disruption in food production
- Sea level will rise causing inundation of coastlines
- Displacement of large numbers of people
- UV radiation will increase
- Further increase in pollution
- Changes in precipitation and temperature patterns
- Limited fresh water supply.

What can be done? Climate change and its associated effect on human health are a global problem. National governments and international organizations are fully aware of the health consequences and try to stem the slide to climatic chaos by discussing possible solutions. The global summits in Rio and Kyoto are a prime example for international cooperation and, unfortunately, also for international incoherence. Heavy air polluters, such as the US and Australia, have not to date ratified the Kyoto protocol. So, why should I care as an individual? Can I make a difference?

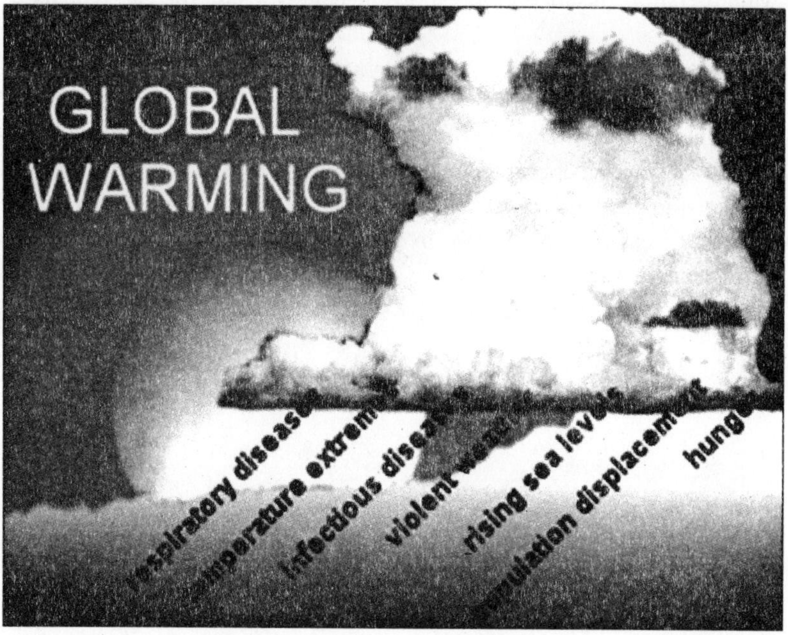

Yes, we can make a difference! We can lobby our local politician and cast our vote accordingly. We can also improve the so-called microclimate—the weather on a small scale, and improve our health in the process. To give you an example from own experience, my wife and I bought a patch of grass, or 'paddock' as we call it here in Australia, on which we built a home. Unfortunately, the only tree on our land fell over and nothing else protected us from the cold winter gales and the hot summer winds. So we planted new trees and shrubs—more than a thousand of them. Only five years later, the microclimate changed significantly for the better. Today the trees slow down the howling winds and adjust the humidity to comfortable levels. And besides the fact that the number of bird species doubled, the trees now limit the impact of temperature extremes.

You don't have to plant thousands of trees, though. Just a few pot plants on your office desk or on your balcony will make a difference. Once the word of the benefits spreads in the neighbourhood, a few plants may grow to thousands of plants on all balconies and in backyards. There are so many ways for us individuals to make a difference: use or buy 'green' energy, drive a car with low fuel consumption, walk the short distance to the shops instead of using the car—the list is endless.

I didn't write this book to tell you about alternative energies and ways to halt global warming. This book is about giving you the awareness that your environment, in this case the weather, has a much greater impact on your wellbeing than any of us would like to admit. If my book succeeds in convincing you of this, then it is only a small step towards the awareness that everything in nature is connected. Care about the environment, care about global warming, care about ozone depletion, and you'll know about the weather and your health.

Bibliography

Weather and health issues cross many fields of science. It is, therefore, no surprise that thousands of articles and reports are spread amongst a variety of print and electronic media. It is beyond the scope of this book to list all related sources. Nevertheless, the following bibliography is extensive enough to point you in the right direction if you want to find further reading material.

Books

Collins, J. F. 1995, *Your Eyes: An Owner's Guide*, Prentice Hall, Englewood Cliffs, NJ.

Colls, K. & Whitaker, R. 1990, *The Australian Weather Book*, Child & Associates Publishing Pty Ltd, Sydney.

Commonwealth Scientific and Industrial Research Organization 1986, *Weather & Climate*, CSIRO Atmospheric Research Programmes, Canberra.

Dyson-Holland, V. 1980, *Meteorology for Pilots*, D-H Training Systems, Newmerella, Australia.

Ewan, C. E., Bryant, E. A., Calvert, G. D. & Garrick, J. A. 1993, *Health in the Greenhouse*, Australian Government Publishing Service, Canberra.

Forsythe, E. 1977, *Asthma, Hay Fever and other Allergies*, Sun Books Pty Ltd, South Melbourne.

Glasspool, M. 1984, *Eyes, their Problems and Treatments*, Methuen Australia Pty Ltd, Sydney, Australia.

Gribbin, J. 1979, *Weather Force*, A P Publishing Pty Ltd, 428 George Street, Sydney.

Gould, H. 1974, *Headaches and Health,* Wren Publishing Pty Ltd, Melbourne.

Lance, J.W. 1998, *Migraine and other Headaches,* Simon & Schuster, 20 Barcoo St, Sydney.

Gribbin, J. 1990, *Hothouse Earth: The Greenhouse Effect & Gaia,* Bantam Press, 61–63 Uxbridge Road, London W5 5SA.

Landsberg, H. E. 1987, 'Something in the Air', *Yearbook of Science and the Future,* Encyclopaedia Britannica Inc., USA.

Larson, E. D. 1996, *Mayo Clinic Family Health Book,* 2nd Edition, William Morrow and Company Inc., New York.

National Health and Medical Research Council 1989, *Health Effects of Ozone Layer Depletion,* Australian Government Publishing Service, Canberra.

Watson, L. 1984, *Heaven's Breath: A Natural History of the Wind,* Hodder and Stoughton Ltd, Mill Road, Kent, UK.

BOOKS OF RELATED INTEREST FROM NAB

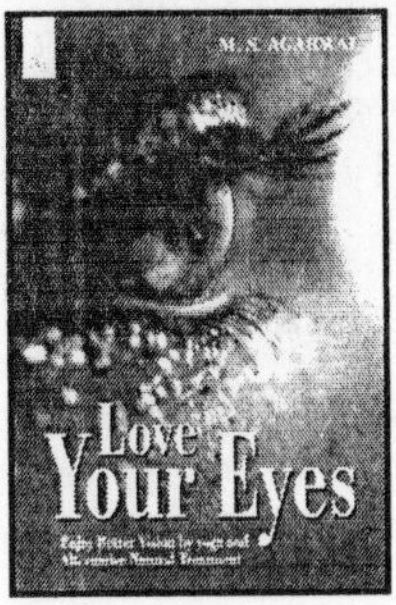

LOVE YOUR EYES —*M.S. Agarwal*
Explaining the details of our beautiful eyes, the book explores their anatomy and functioning. It is a must read for those searching complete knowledge about the gift of sight and alternative treatment for related disorders.

ISBN: 978-81-7822-319-3

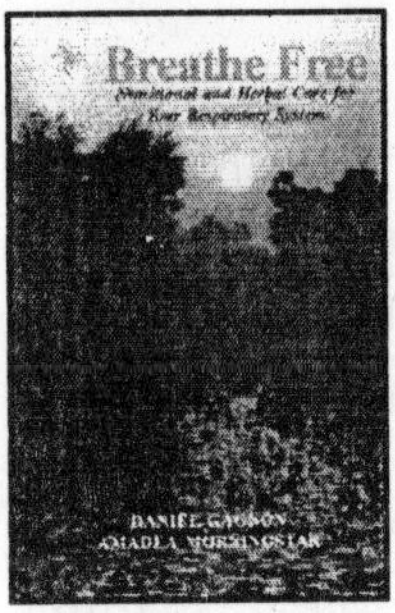

BREATHE FREE: Nutritional and Herbal Care for Your Respiratory System—*Daniel Gagnon and Amadea Morningstar*
It provides therapeutic guidelines for holistic approach and an expose on respiratory diseases and their natural treatment.

ISBN: 978-81-7822-018-5

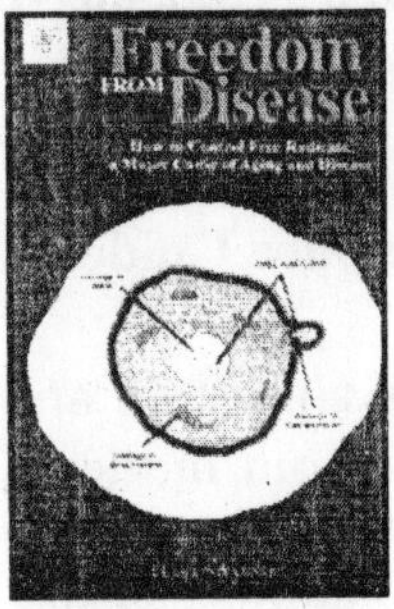

FREEDOM FROM DISEASE: How to Control Free Radicals, a Major Cause of Aging and Disease—*Hari Sharma*
With the help of this book you will find how free radicals are implicated in everything from heart attacks to wrinkled skin, from cataracts to cancer. Learn how the body fights free radicals with its powerful enzyme army—how it desperately needs reinforcement—and why vitamins and drugs are far too weak to fill the gap.

ISBN: 978-81-7822-224-0

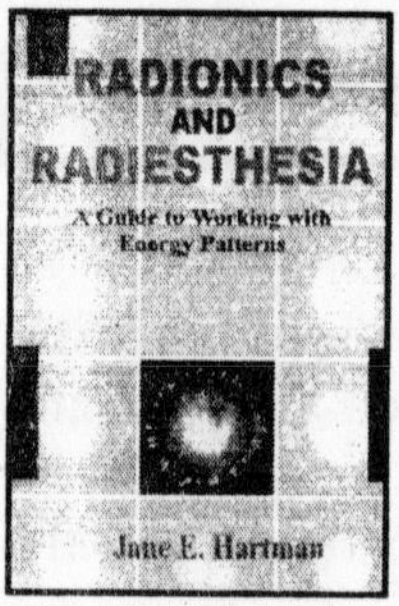

RADIONICS AND RADIESTHESIA: A Guide to Working with Energy Patterns— *Jane E. Hartman*

Everything that exists, including thought, is a form of energy. Such as the wisdom guiding the increasingly widespread practice of radionics (healing at a distance) and its complement radiesthesia (dowsing).

ISBN: 978-81-7822-166-3

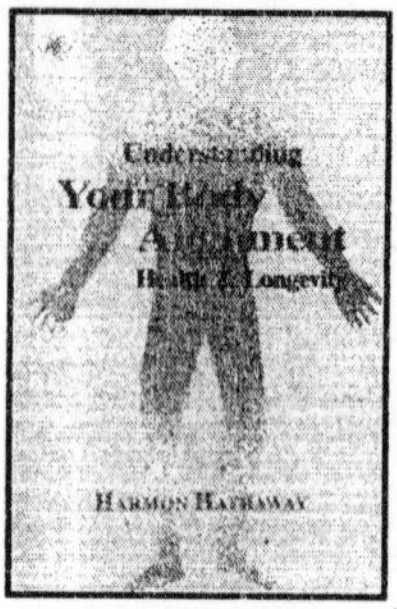

UNDERSTANDING YOUR BODY ALIGNMENT: Health and Longevity — *Harmon Hathaway*

The book offers very effective techniques for releasing tension and frozen energy, helping the body to function fully. It helps to reach the sacred point of confluence of mind, body and spirit in holistic perspective.

It can provide a direct natural solution to many human illnesses, especially those related to: Emphysema, Asthma, Lung diseases, Bursitis, Tendonitis and Arthritis, etc.

ISBN: 978-81-7822-001-7

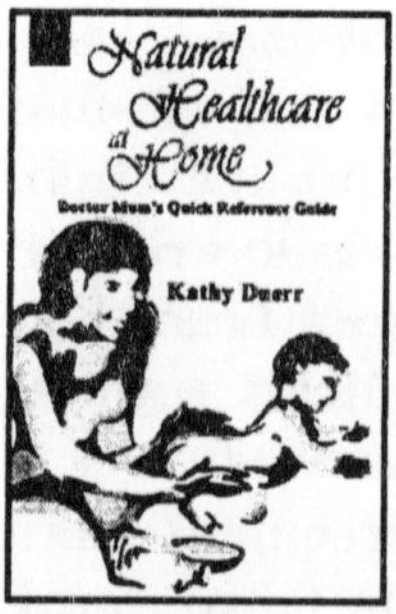

NATURAL HEALTHCARE AT HOME: Doctor Mum's Quick Reference Guide — *Kathy Duerr*

Natural Healthcare at Home is a must for any home with small children. In our modern-day, quick-fix world we have come to rely heavily on antibiotics and chemical drugs which can suppress the immune system and subject our children to short-term side-effects and long-term consequences.

ISBN: 978-81-7822-017-8